D0909157

Please Don't
Feed the
Daisy

Living, Loving,

and

Losing Weight

with the

World's Hungriest Dog

HYPERION
• • • • •
NEW YORK

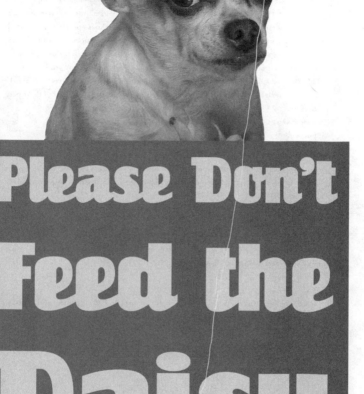

Please Don't Feed the Daisy

Beverly West AND **Jason Bergund**

EAST BATON ROUGE PARISH LIBRARY
7711 GOODWOOD BOULEVARD
BATON ROUGE, LOUISIANA 70806

Note to Reader: Please note this book contains a personal account of the authors' relationship with their pets and is not intended to replace the advice of a veterinarian. All matters regarding the health of your pets, including any pregnancies or diets, require professional supervision. Consult your veterinarian before adopting the suggestions in this book. None of the material in this book should be used as a substitute for veterinarian care and treatment. While the authors specify certain products that they used for their pets with good results, the authors' inclusion of the products in no way represents an endorsement by the Publisher, nor does the exclusion of a product or trade name represent a negative judgment of any kind.

The Authors and Publisher disclaim any liability directly or indirectly from the use of the material in this book by any person, or by any person on behalf of their pet.

Copyright © 2009 Beverly and Jason Bergund
All photographs by Jason Bergund

All rights reserved. No part of this book may be used or reproduced in any manner whatsoever without the written permission of the Publisher. Printed in the United States of America. For information address Hyperion, 114 Fifth Avenue, New York, New York 10011.

Library of Congress Cataloging-in-Publication Data

West, Beverly.
    Please don't feed the Daisy : living, loving, and losing weight with the world's hungriest dog / Beverly West and Jason Bergund.
        p. cm.
    ISBN 978-1-4013-2337-0
1. Health. 2. Reducing diet. 3. Pets—Therapeutic use. 4. Pets—Feeding and feeds. 5. Human-animal relationships. 6. Chihuahua (Dog breed). 7. Pug. I. Bergund, Jason. II. Title.
    RA776.W466 2009
    613.2'5—dc22
        2008052943

Hyperion books are available for special promotions and premiums. For details contact the HarperCollins Special Markets Department in the New York office at 212-207-7528, fax 212-207-7222, or email spsales@harpercollins.com.

Design by Sunil Manchikanti

FIRST EDITION
10 9 8 7 6 5 4 3 2 1

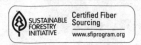

SUSTAINABLE FORESTRY INITIATIVE
Certified Fiber Sourcing
www.sfiprogram.org

THIS LABEL APPLIES TO TEXT STOCK

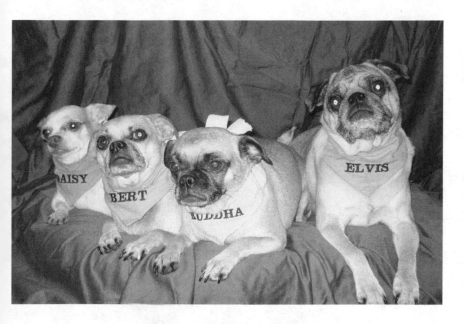

To our fat Daisy and Daisys
everywhere, who remind us
every day that love comes in
all shapes, colors, and sizes.

Acknowledgments

Bev and Jason would like to thank our talented and inspiring editors, Gretchen Young and Elizabeth Sabo, for their enthusiasm, insight, and support. Thanks also to Anne Newgarden for the world-class copyedit and to Sunil Manchikanti for the enchanting book design.

A very special thanks to our agent Jenny Bent, who remains the undisputed queen of all agents as well as a dear friend, and to our menagerie of pets, who remind us every day of the power of unconditional love.

Thanks also to our family and friends, Pamela Eisermann, Kristopher Monroe, Gretchen Krull, Kim Doi, Deborah Jean Baynes, Ellen Rees, David Olds, Susan Coates, Colette Linnihan, John and Darlene Bergund, Stella Holden, Joe Kolker, and Suzanne Polinski for her talent and handiwork on the great puppy costumes (www.missdaphnes.com). Thanks also to our divinely inspired vet Kim Rosenthal at West Side Veterinary Center in New York City, who set us all on a healthier path. And thanks to Dov Treiman, Carolyn Rualo, Bill Geller, Christopher Halligan, and Adam Leitman Bailey, our unsung heroes.

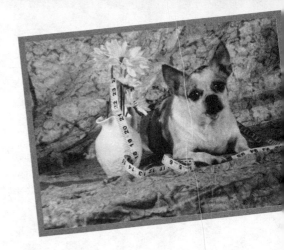

Contents

Please Don't Feed the Daisy

Love, Food, and Dogs

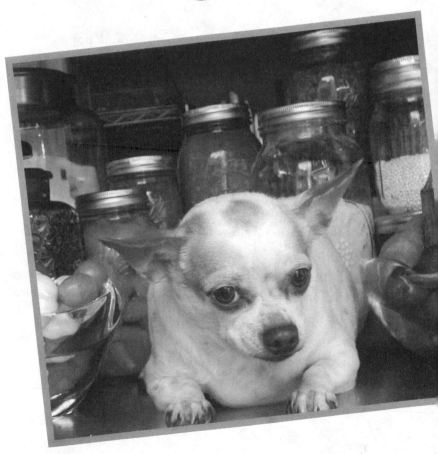

Falling in love, a great meal, and puppies are life's showstoppers. They're God forcing us to pay attention. In their presence, you aren't thinking about anything except *How wonderful! How delicious! How cute!* For that instant, there's no past, no future, no causes or consequences, no puddle in the hallway or number on the scale, no bottom line. There's only the uncomplicated enjoyment of the here and now. You string a few months of moments like this together, and you'll be surprised where you wind up.

Which I guess is how I find myself now, at the age of forty-seven, living with four dogs, one cat, two turtles, and fifteen fish in a one-bedroom apartment in New York City, married to a man seventeen years younger than me. And I've never been happier.

Of course, this isn't at all the life I expected.

I'm not exactly sure what I had in mind for myself, but I'm pretty sure that whatever it was involved fewer dogs. Probably a bigger apartment, too, and I'm certain a smaller waistline. But I love how life is mysterious like that. It never brings what you expect, and yet manages to deliver exactly what you need, whether or not you know it at the time.

When Jason and the dogs came along, mostly what it felt like was a whole lot of chaos coupled with an alarming lack of shelf space. But as our puppies grew into dogs, and eventually had puppies themselves, Jason and I, quite unbeknownst to ourselves, were building a home and a family of our own. What I've come to realize is that what initially felt like the world falling apart was actually just the growing pains of a new and better one being born.

This is the story of our family's adventure with love, food, and dogs, all of which have taught us some very important lifelong lessons, like how to go with the flow, how to trust the unknown, and how to have faith in the recipes of life. We've learned that mistakes create some fabulous taste treats, that we can draw healthy boundaries and maintain them, and that we can make and sustain the changes that we want to make in ourselves, our bodies, and our lives. And most importantly, we've learned to spend as much time as possible appreciating the small moments and the smaller portions of life, and counting our blessings along with our calories, four dogs, one cat, two turtles, and fifteen fish at a time.

One

How Much Is That
Daisy
in the Window?

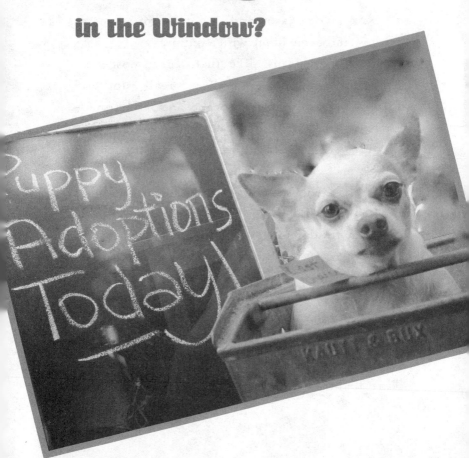

One day, Jason and I went out for a cheese-burger, and came home with a puppy.

It happened just like that. Like most life-changing events do. And when I really stop and think about it now, it was probably one of the stupidest ideas we'd ever had. Although it's a good thing we didn't realize it then, because it also turned out to be one of our finest hours.

And of course, you have to forgive yourself during times like these. In the aftermath of a sudden and fundamental shift in business as usual, like 9/11 was in New York City, most of us felt apart and aside from everyday life for a while. It was as if everything stopped, life held its breath, and everybody just waited to see what the lay of the land would be like once the dust settled. Until then, the regular rules and regulations of life just didn't apply. This included the rules and regulations about regular exercise, smoking, trans fats, anti-anxiety meds, alternate-side-of-the-street parking, drinking, romance, and puppies, to name just a few.

I suspect that Jason had a pretty good idea of what was going to happen that day, but I, as usual, was only thinking about the next fry fix. In the toxic dust and confusion that plumed perpetually from downtown Manhattan in those weeks and months following 9/11, carb-depleting had lost all of its appeal, and I didn't want to eat anything unless it was battered and fried.

"I think there's a diner on the next block that has *fabulous* onion rings," said Jason, and grinned at me that way he does. Jason always did know just how to get to me. And being a native son of Ohio, Jason knew from onion rings. There was no way I was going to ignore a recommendation of his in that department. He was a true connoisseur. And then he said coyly, "I think there's a pet store right next door. And I think it's adoption day. Can we go look at the puppies, pleeeaaasse?"

I rolled my eyes, but of course I was going to say yes. I could never say no to Jason, not since the day I'd met him three years before. He was a nineteen-year-old dancer/barista back then, but I'm pretty sure he'd lied and told me he was twenty. Not that this was much of a distinction, since he still wasn't old enough to get into a bar . . . although this never seemed to stop him. Jason was and is unusually poised for his age. And even back then, except for the times when he was wearing a plastic shirt and had glued rhinestones on his eyes, he looked almost legal.

I, on the other hand, was a thirty-six-year-old author then, and I'm pretty sure I told him that, but somehow this didn't seem to matter. From the moment our eyes met over an avenue full of Macy's floats and a platter piled high with questionable-looking lox at that infamous Thanksgiving Day Parade brunch, we'd been inseparable. It was one of the many cosmic imponderables that would come to characterize our relationship. There were a million reasons why we shouldn't fit, and yet, for some reason, we did.

Here we are on the day that we met (see next page).

Those drinks we have in our hands were really good, although as you can see, they are both almost gone. We had about four or five of those theme concoctions that afternoon in order to chase that indigestible lox. Jason figured out how to make them and we drink them every Thanksgiving now.

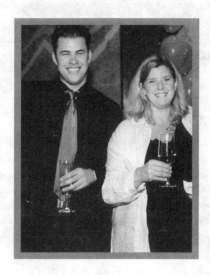

Jason calls them Macy's Day Floats. Take one out for a test drive the next time you're in the mood to defy gravity.

"All right, we can go by the pet store, but if it is adoption day, we are just *looking*," I told him. I knew Jason really wanted a dog. I knew because he'd managed to work the word *puppy* into every other sentence for the last month and a half. Jason had lost his dog in the fallout, and since then he'd been as obsessed with getting a puppy as I was with french fries. Jason had also lost his apartment, and since I was going through a divorce myself, Jason had been "staying with me" until we both found our way back onto the road we had been traveling before things

The Macy's Day Float

HERE'S WHAT YOU'LL NEED:
1 ounce vodka
Splash Framboise
3 ounces champagne
Fresh red raspberries

HERE'S HOW YOU DO IT: Pour vodka and Framboise into the bottom of a very expensive-looking champagne flute. Fill to the top with champagne and garnish with 1 fresh raspberry. Repeat until you are hovering at least 25 feet above the treetops. Maintain a lower altitude if you are experiencing wind gusts over 40 mph.

got so weird. We were on an extended detour, we figured, and eventually, we'd find our way back onto the main highway. In the meantime, at least as far as I was concerned, a dog was out of the question. There just wasn't room for me, Jason, all of Jason's stuff that wouldn't fit in storage, including his sweeping epic of a media collection, *and* a dog in my junior one-bedroom. We could barely breathe as it was. And besides, I was a cat person.

When we finally reached the pet store, Jason pushed his face against the glass to get a better look at the rescue puppies that were up for adoption. There weren't many to choose from that day. There were three anxious-looking Yorkies whose nerves would never tolerate the rough-and-tumble life-style of our party pad. Wrestling with each other right in front were two poodles, and I knew we were safe there because Jason is a poodleist, and therefore discriminated against poodles. And tucked back in the far corner was one nondescript and not particularly adorable white Chihuahua puppy with a heart-shaped spot on her butt and a broken tail, who looked like she'd just been marked down for clearance. Now, I'm not sure why what happened next happened. I had a pretty clean shot at a puppyless exit at this point, but for some reason, I didn't take it.

Instead I said, "Oh Jason, look at that cute little white one."

It wasn't that this Chihuahua puppy was particularly cute, because to be perfectly honest, she wasn't. She looked like a full-grown dog, only smaller. She was clearly an old soul. And it was obvious that she'd been in the window for a while. She was used to being on display, and used to being regularly passed over. Well, there were a lot of homeless dogs in the wake of 9/11, so she had a lot of competition. But she had this look that seemed to say, "So maybe my stocks have momentarily plunged, but *whatever*, I'm a bitch and I know what I'm worth." From the minute I looked into her eyes, I was a total goner, and Jason, being Jason, picked up on it immediately.

"Should we go in and ask if we can hold her?" said Jason. Granted, this inscrutable little ghetto Chihuahua was not the adorable pug he'd been dreaming of, but bottom line, Jason wanted a puppy. Like I said, Jason is a shrewd man, despite his years. He moved to New York all by himself at seventeen, and this had taught him very young that when chances like this come along, you take them without asking too many questions.

"Can we hold the little white puppy?" Jason asked an overjoyed volunteer, who pulled the puppy immediately out of the window and thrust her into my arms. The puppy cuddled into the crook of my neck and stuck a cold nose, followed by a startlingly long tongue, up my left nostril. You think I'm kidding? Just take a look at the length of this thing. It's seriously supernatural.

"Awww," said Jason. "She loves you."

"Awww," said the clerk, who I think at this point was almost jumping up and down at the thought of this peculiar white puppy finding a home. "She's been waiting for you two for a long time. We were

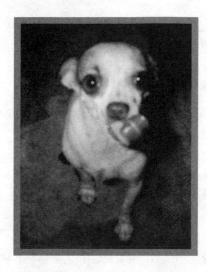

just about to take her out of the window. But something told me to leave her in just one more day."

I really didn't want to know what "take her out of the window" meant. Obviously, neither did Jason, because before I managed to get the puppy's tongue out of my nose, he had already picked out a lavender sweater with a big pearl button on it, and pulled out his wallet.

"I think we should call her Daisy," said Jason matter-of-factly. "Daisies *are* the friendliest flower."

Daisy worked for me. And it seemed to work for Daisy, who had fallen asleep and virtually disappeared into her purple cable-knit behind that enormous pearl button. Jason put her in my arms. Oh my God, I was a middle-aged divorcee holding a little dog in a sweater. I was *that* woman. How did this happen?

Jason grabbed the food and the wee-wee pads, and the twelve different little toys and treats, and the three additional sweaters, and the princess bed he'd slipped in while I wasn't looking, and dragged me out to hail a cab before I could change my mind. Not that I could have, at that point. Once I grab on to something, I very rarely let go.

Daisy sat quietly in my lap on the cab ride home, watching her new world fly by for the first time through a cab window. Looking down at Daisy, so utterly at peace with whatever was going to happen next, I realized that for the first time since that terrible day just over a month before, I had gone at least thirty minutes and twenty seconds without even once thinking about an onion ring or a single french fry.

Learning to Feed the Daisy

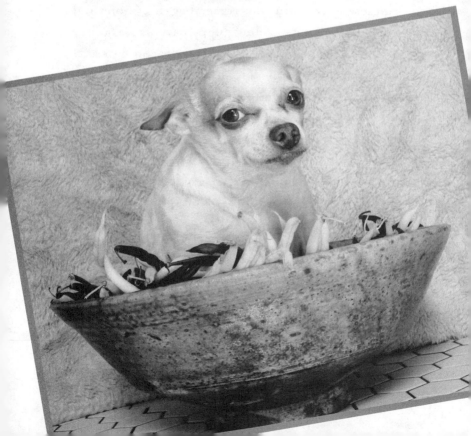

Looking at Daisy now, and trying without success to wrap my fingers around her current circumference, it's funny to remember that Jason's and my first challenge as new puppy parents was to try and get her to eat something. Her response to sudden transition seemed to have been the opposite of mine. While my circular obsessive thoughts always revolved around the next empty calorie, Daisy seemed to find solace in turning up her nose at every morsel of puppy comfort food we offered her. And we worried about her, because she looked so, I don't know, pathetic. I mean, look at her.

And it's not like she looked any bigger when she was dry. She had hardly any fur. So I desperately wanted to put some meat on her bones. But Daisy wasn't interested. She just sat quietly on the couch, all two and half pounds of her, curled into a tiny crook in a nearby pillow, and gazed at us, immovable.

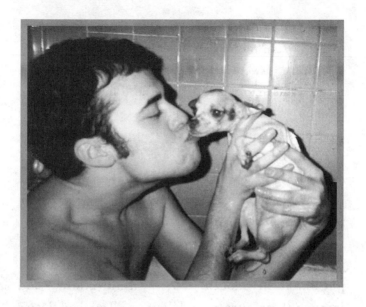

Meanwhile, Jason and I frantically waved every over-priced treat we'd brought home from the pet store in her face. But neither the Greenies biscuit, nor the teeny tiny rawhide shoe, nor the Pup-Peroni, nor even the Yummy Chummies seemed to impress her in the slightest.

It's not that she was particularly cranky or disagreeable about it. She simply refused to be tempted, and I began to wonder if that look in her eye, which I had interpreted as doggie wisdom at the pet store, was in fact something else altogether . . . something that might come into play when we tried to get her to do other things, too, like poop on a pad, for example. Or sit.

"Well, just because she's not going to eat doesn't mean we have to starve," I said, and headed into the kitchen. "Besides, I baked a cake. We can't exactly have dessert without a meal." I admit it. I was a little put out. I'm a passionate cook, I take my calories seriously, and it was hard not to take culinary rejection like this personally, even if it was from a forty-two-ounce Chihuahua.

"Dinner sounds good, doesn't it, Daisy?" said Jason, who broke open a fresh pack of Smackos and put one in his mouth. "*Mmmm*-mmm-mmm," said Jason, "these sure are delicious. Too bad Daisy can't have any." Daisy buried her head in the couch pillow. Well, there was a reason that Jason's résumé said dancer/actor, rather than actor/dancer. Daisy wasn't buying his performance for a second. And even I had to admit, that *fakon* looked awful.

"Maybe she's like me," I said, picking out a couple of choice Idaho's finest and starting to slice them into matchsticks. "Maybe she only wants to eat french fries." Well, it made sense to me at the time. I was writing my cookbook and was deep into the chapter on comfort food. In fact, I had been deep into my chapter on comfort food for the last four months. And while this kind of singular creative focus did not do wonders for my deadline or my waistline, I did get a chance to polish each and every mushy beige, salty, and sweet delicacy I'd come up with to absolute perfection. I felt really absolutely solid about my Change Your World Chocolate Chip Cookie à la Mode, my Empathy Éclairs, and my Somebody Loves You Smashed Potatoes, but the exact formula for Comfort Fries continued to elude me. Finally, though, I believed I had come up with *the* recipe for the world's most perfectly crisped french fry, but before I could be sure, I needed to do the Jason test. If I saw that look on his face that let me know he was feeling the spud love, I'd know I had finally connected. His smile was my final authority. The recipe is on the next page by the way, for the next time you want a little deep fried lovin' with your salt and ketchup.

"I defy anybody, two legs or four, to say no to these puppies," I said, holding up one perfectly prepared french fry. "Now where is that picky pooch?"

I put the fry next to her and stood back and waited for her to weaken. Of course, she didn't

Comfort Fries

HERE'S WHAT YOU'LL NEED:

Large Idaho potatoes (as many as you can
    slice without flirting with carpal
    tunnel syndrome)
4 tablespoons confectioners' sugar
3 tablespoons fresh lemon juice
4 cups cold water
3 cups canola oil
A lot of salt
A lot of ketchup
Mayonnaise and butter optional

HERE'S HOW YOU DO IT: Cut your potatoes into thin matchsticks. Dissolve confectioners' sugar in lemon juice and water and soak your fries for as long as you can stand it. Heat your oil to 350°F. Drain your potatoes thoroughly, pat dry with a towel, then submerge in the oil. And for God's sake, don't overcrowd the pan. When they are golden brown, remove them from the oil and drain on paper towels. Toss with salt, and serve immediately with ketchup, salt, mayonnaise, butter, etc. Repeat process as often as necessary.

want those nasty old doggie treats, I thought. What do they make them out of, anyway, pig snouts and gorilla knuckles? But wait until she got a load of *my* cooking. Daisy moved cautiously closer to the french fry.

"She moved!" said Jason.

"Shhh," I said, "don't scare her."

After the most pregnant of pauses, Daisy stretched forward and gave a tentative sniff, then pushed my perfect french fry resolutely off the couch and onto the floor.

We both looked crushed. This latest act of puppy rebellion was bordering on blasphemy. In our new and tentative household, dinner had become more than a meal; it was a religion, and we were very devout. Our days were organized around our nightly ritual. In the morning, we would come up with a menu that suited our mood and our budget, both of which fluctuated profoundly at the time. Then we would venture out in search of the black walnuts, white truffle oil, creamy Camembert, or the Manwich sauce we needed. Then, when evening finally fell, Jason and I would cook like there was no tomorrow until our ragtag band of semi-inebriated and hungry pilgrims would show up to sample the fare. Our biggest turnout was always Life Is Sweeter with Sauce Lasagna night. Well, I do make a mean red sauce. You'll find the recipe on the next page. You can try it out the next time you're in the mood to inspire a little undying gratitude among your personal congregation.

Life Is Sweeter with Sauce Lasagna

FOR THE MEAT SAUCE:
1 Vidalia onion, minced
2 tablespoons extra virgin
    olive oil
1 pound sweet Italian sausage
1 pound hot Italian sausage
1 small can tomato paste
1/2 cup good red wine
Two 15-ounce cans tomato puree
1 tablespoon sugar
1 Parmigiano Regiano rind or 3 table-
    spoons grated Parmesan
Salt and pepper to taste
2 teaspoons dried oregano or
    2 tablespoons fresh oregano
1 teaspoon dried basil or 2 tablespoons
    fresh basil
1 pound ground beef

HERE'S HOW YOU DO IT: Sauté minced onion in olive oil until clear. Add sausages and sauté until browned. Reduce heat slightly, add tomato paste, and allow to simmer until it forms a light crust on the bottom of the pan. Next, deglaze with the red wine, and scrape up the crust off the bottom of the pan to form the base of your sauce. Add tomato puree, sugar, cheese, salt, and spices. Finally, break up the ground beef and toss into the sauce. Cover and simmer on low for at least 2 hours.

FOR THE FILLING:
1 pound fresh ricotta cheese
2 large eggs

(Continued)

1 1/2 teaspoons fresh oregano, basil, and
   parsley (half the amount if dried)
Dash extra virgin olive oil
1/2 pound fresh mozzarella

Cream all ingredients except the mozzarella together until you have formed a smooth paste. Then fold in grated mozzarella.

TO MAKE THE LASAGNA:
1 pound lasagna noodles
2 to 3 cups meat sauce
2 to 3 cups filling
1/2 pound mozzarella cheese
1/2 cup grated Parmesan

HERE'S HOW YOU DO IT: Preheat oven to 375°F. Soak 1 pound of lasagna noodles in very hot water. Put a thin coating of sauce on the bottom of a 9 × 11 baking pan. Place a single layer of noodles on the bottom of the pan, cover completely with the sauce, and then cover with a layer of the filling (ricotta cheese) mixture and a thin layer of mozzarella and Parmesan. Cover with sausage and more sauce. Repeat process for three layers total, then finish with remaining mozzarella and Parmesan and bake for 30 to 40 minutes until cheese on the top is nicely browned. Let stand for 10 to 15 minutes before serving. Then dive in with both hands, and consider bibs, because sometimes the sauce really flies when you put this dish on the table.

On the next page is Jason's sauce for the night.

So, needless to say, in a pasta-rich, sauce-infused, pear-happy atmosphere like this one, turning up your nose at something as sacred as the world's most perfect french fry was simply not done.

Pear Jason

HERE'S WHAT YOU'LL NEED:
Poire Williams pear brandy
Pear juice (preferably fresh)
A good champagne or sparkling wine

HERE'S HOW YOU DO IT: Pour 2 dashes of the Poire Williams into your favorite flutes, along with 2 dashes of pear juice. If you prefer your cocktails sweeter, feel free to add more pear juice. Pop your champagne and pour over the pear mixture, and enjoy!

I began to wonder if Jason and I had inadvertently adopted a heretic into our midst.

"Maybe it's just too hot," said Jason helplessly. I was still staring at the fry on the ground in disbelief. This dog had been living on water and baked by-products for God's sake, and she hadn't eaten anything at all in hours. How could she say no to people food? It was almost . . . undoggylike.

I looked at Daisy, trying to read the meaning behind her passive resistance. But all I saw was that same inscrutable look of acceptance mixed with resolve that I'd seen in the pet store window. She was a stubborn enigma, that's for sure.

"Why don't we try this?" Jason said, as he emerged

from the bowels of the fridge with something green in his hand. It was a tin of edemame beans left over from the weekend's Japanese takeout. True to form, the only thing we had left over was the roughage.

"She's not going to eat that," I said, horrified. "It's a, I mean, it's a . . . vegetable! Dogs don't eat vegetables."

"Actually," said Jason, "it's a legume." And as soon as he held it out to Daisy, she inhaled the bean and licked her lips, and for the first time since we'd brought her home, looked actually intrigued. Maybe it's a fluke, I thought. Maybe she got confused and thought the edemame was something else, like bacon. But no sooner had I formed that comforting thought when Jason held out another fresh shiny bean and Daisy gobbled it down and got up and wagged her tail and begged for another one.

And then Jason flashed me that smile, and I swear, so did Daisy. And in that moment, I knew in my gut the way that you do, that quite unexpectedly and mysteriously, the time had come to move on to my next chapter. And clearly, the new chapter was going to include some roughage.

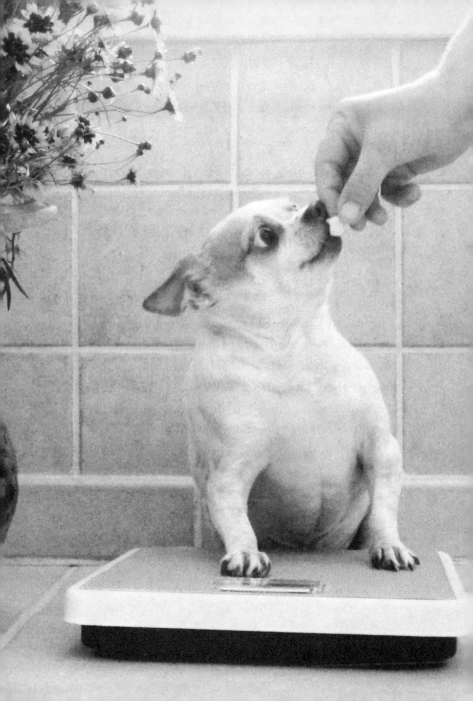

Healthy Treats for Picky Pooches

Flossies by Merrick (they come in small, medium, and large sizes): Dogs *love* them, and because of their shape, they are great for your dog's teeth, too! Due to their sudden trendy status, Flossies have gotten a little pricey, but for an every-once-in-a-while puppy treat extravaganza, they're excellent. These bones are also remarkably resilient, so it's two hours of pure puppy decadence.

Vitality treats by Dogswell: These delicious chicken treats come in a variety of flavors, and all with their unique supplement additives to provide homeopathic support for a variety of concerns. For example, they have Happy Hips with glucosamine and chondroitin to promote joint health, and Breathies to sweeten your dog's breath and promote upper respiratory health. You get the idea. It's a treat but it's a supplement but it's a treat.

WildSide Salmon treats from the WildSide Salmon Company: Our dogs do go wild for these freeze-dried salmon treats—actually so does our cat—and they are not only delicious and nutritious, but good for the environment. Salmon fished in Alaska for roe used to be ground up, then dumped back into Alaskan bays and inlets. Today the WildSide Salmon Company makes a delicious and healthful treat for our dogs with this wonderful protein instead of tossing it away to pollute our waters.

Filly's Canine Cookies: These delicious handmade treats began as

(Continued)

a student project by Filly Mastrangelo at the Life Experience School, a place for individuals with special needs in Millis, Massachusetts. Portions of the proceeds are donated to various charitable organizations, including those for autism research and the care of stray animals (www.fillyscaninecookies.com).

Three

Yours, Mine, and Ours

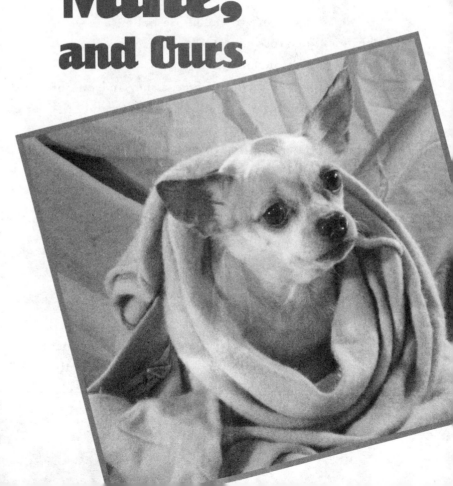

Daisy wasn't in the house but a week when the question arose about who Daisy actually belonged to. Was she Jason's dog? Was she mine? Was she ours? It was a complicated issue, and one of those questions that begged about a thousand others. It was like pulling a string on a hand-knitted afghan. If you tug on it hard enough the whole weave loosens, and after a while the blanket just doesn't keep you warm anymore.

Originally, Daisy was intended to be Jason's dog. He was the one with the puppy-mania. This made it tough for me, though, during those long mornings when Jason was away at work and I was home alone with Daisy. I'd sit at my desk and write while Daisy sat on the couch staring at me.

I knew that I should probably pick her up and hold her in my lap. She looked so small and vulnerable over there all by herself on that great big couch. But for some reason I just couldn't. She was so cute and so tiny, but she was also somebody else's dog. When the day came for Jason to move out, Daisy was going with him, and this made me a little reluctant to get too attached. It was going to be hard enough to let Jason go. I didn't want to throw a scene straight out of *Old Yeller* into the mix. So I kept my distance. Better safe than sorry.

As usual, though, my attempts at self-preservation lasted about forty-eight hours, and then caution went straight into the wind's eye. It started slowly, as these things do. First, Daisy learned to jump off the couch, and then she'd trot over to me, and before I knew it she was curled at my feet and staring up at me with a look that said, "You know you want it."

And she was right. I did. And sure enough, before long Daisy was off the floor and curled up in my lap like she'd been there all along. I was trying very hard to work, but mostly I was instant messaging with Jason, watching trash TV, and counting the minutes until six o'clock. After 9/11, even though I was a writer, it was hard to know what to say for a while. It was like living in giant ellipses. So mostly, Daisy and I spent our days wrapped up in my baby blue cashmere shawl, just waiting patiently together for Jason to finally come home. And of course in the process, while neither one of us was really noticing, Daisy and I were falling madly in love.

Pretty soon, I got so used to having Daisy by my side that it felt like something was missing when I put her down and went into the test kitchen in the afternoons to try out the recipes I'd written that day. Daisy, as usual, found a way to solve the problem more quickly than I did. I was working on my Food for Thought chapter, which featured foods that were designed to inspire and enlighten. I was feeling optimistic again with a new puppy in the house. And I'd taken the edamame as an omen and was trying to introduce a little green into our routine. This day, I was working on my Get Your Motor Running Green Chile, a concoction so deliciously spicy that it was guaranteed to put the tiger back in anybody's tank. It was green all right, but something was missing. I couldn't put my finger on it. I was making an effort to cook light, so today was all about finding that extra something special that would make my chile sing like a strolling mariachi band, only without three tablespoons of lard. It's amazing to discover how absolutely essential pork rendering can be at certain moments.

While I was trying to puzzle out a substitute for trans fats, which is never easy, I looked over for Daisy, who I had thought was curled up in her usual place on the kitchen rug, snoozing in a tiny beam of sunlight.

But Daisy wasn't there. Terror struck. I put down the garlic and went frantically in search of her, petrified that my old cat Nick had finally seized his moment. He'd been licking his chops and staring at her menacingly ever since we'd brought her home. He was subtle about it, and Daisy was oblivious, but I knew it was there. Can't you tell he's just biding his time?

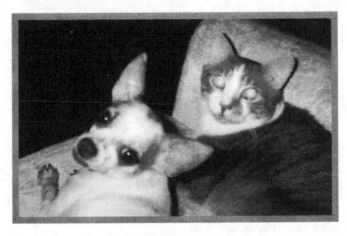

Fortunately, I found Nick snoozing benignly by the radiator, unconcerned with the affairs of mice and dogs, as he had been for the majority of the last thirteen years. Thank God some things never change. But there was no sign of Daisy. She was so tiny, and the apartment was still a maze of unalphabetized videos and CDs, mismatched dance shoes, disassembled Metro Shelves, books, old *Playbills*, more books, Bette Midler posters, and a mountain of Jason's club clothes. I might never find her amidst the rubble of our past lives.

Then I heard a small rustling in my office, and Daisy emerged, dragging my baby blue cashmere shawl behind her. The shawl was at least five times her length and twice as wide. It trailed behind her like a long, fuzzy blue kite. I could tell that it was taking every ounce of her strength and then some to tug that enormous wrap through the living room, but she went at it with such focus, such single-minded determination, that she overcame the laws of physics cheerfully, and deposited the shawl in a cuddly heap at my feet. Then she looked up at me, triumphant, and wagged her tail.

"Awww," I said, touched at the sheer scale of her gesture. "I love you, too, Daisy, but I can't come sit with you. I have work to do."

"Arf," said Daisy.

"I'll sit with you later, once I finish the chile. We'll watch *Judge Judy*."

"Arf, Arf, Arf AARF!!!," said Daisy, starting to get a little annoyed with me. Like I was too slow on the uptake, and I should quit being such a dullard already. I seriously felt like I was in a *Lassie* episode, only I didn't know the lines. What would Timmy do?

And then, finally, I saw the light. I tied the scarf in a knot and slung it across my shoulder, and settled Daisy into the crook of the makeshift pooch pouch. She settled into the blue softness with a sigh and closed her eyes. And then I went back to crushing garlic and roasting peppers while Daisy snoozed at my side. And when it was done, and I tasted the rich broth, I realized that perhaps Daisy had been the missing ingredient all along, because sure enough, the chile was singing. The recipe is on the next page so you can cook up a batch of this liquid gold the next time you're in the mood to find God on a tortilla chip.

"What's cookin' good lookin'?" I looked up from the pot and Jason was home. Six o'clock had come without my having counted the minutes, for once.

"God, I'm Glad You're Home Green Chile," I said, and dipped in a spoon to give Jason a taste.

Daisy's Get Up and Go Green Chile

Preheat oven to 425 degrees F.

HERE'S WHAT YOU'LL NEED:
4 anaheim peppers
4 poblano peppers
4 jalapeño peppers
2 Vidalia onions
2 bulbs of garlic
6 tomatillos
1/2 cup chicken stock
2 tablespoons cilantro
3 tablespoons olive oil
1 tablespoon oregano
1 bay leaf
Juice of 1 lime
Salt and pepper to taste

HERE'S HOW YOU DO IT: Roast the peppers, whole unpeeled onions, whole unpeeled garlic, and whole unpeeled tomatillos at 425 degrees F for about 20 to 25 minutes, then turn them and roast for another 15 to 20 minutes, or 35 to 45 minutes total. Remove from the oven and place in paper sacks. Close the paper bags and allow the peppers, onions, etc. to steam for an hour. Then remove skins and seeds and place in a food processor, add chicken stock and cilantro, and pulse until blended but still slightly chunky. Heat olive oil in a large pan, add the pepper and onion puree, along with oregano, bay leaf, lime juice, salt, and pepper and simmer on low for 20 to 30 minutes. Serve over burritos or tacos, or add pork and serve as a stew. Poach eggs in it. Serve cold as a salsa with chips. Get creative, and use liberally. This sauce is like green ketchup for the soul. Best prepared with a toy Chihuahua hanging on your shoulder.

"Mmm . . . ," said Jason, smacking his lips. And then he saw Daisy hanging from my hip in her cashmere hammock and pointed dramatically, spilling a little of his panacea on his shirt in his amusement. "What is this?" he asked and smirked at me. "A doggy Björn? I think somebody's becoming a puppy person."

"I just didn't want Nick to eat her," I said, trying hard not to sound like the card-carrying, baby-talking, puppy-sweater-and-matching-satchel-buying weird dog person that I now was. "And I'm always afraid I'll step on her, or lose her in this mess."

"Listen," said Jason then, coming into the kitchen, kissing me on the cheek, and dipping yet another chip into my chile. "I've been thinking about it and I think Daisy should be your dog."

"No, don't be ridiculous," I said, slapping his hand out of the pot as he went in for a double dip. "I don't need a Chihuahua, and besides, we got her for you."

"You two are a good fit. Daisy should stay here, no matter what happens. End of discussion. Although of course," Jason added casually over his shoulder as he headed off to change, "this means we need to get another puppy, for me."

Four

Elvis
Enters the
Building

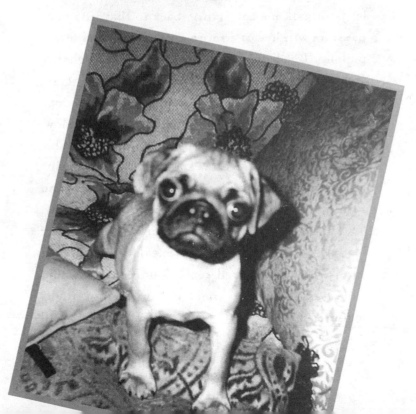

I didn't fall off the Petco truck yesterday, and it's hard enough to fool me once, let alone twice, so it's difficult to imagine in retrospect why I let Jason talk me into going back to that infamous pet store window one more time, just to *look* at the puppies. But I did. We of course, quite by chance according to Jason's recollection, of which I am suspect to this day, chose another rescue pet adoption day to just *look* at the puppies in the window. And there, just *looking* at us, was *the* most adorable apricot pug with an ice-cream-cone tail, long, gangly legs, paws that were way too big for his body, and a smushy pug face that melted our hearts instantly.

I asked the animal rescue volunteer in a rather loudish voice if it were indeed true that pugs snorted incessantly, and snored really loudly at night, and were just generally sneezing, wheezing, high-maintenance beasts that should be avoided at all costs. The puppy chose that precise moment to snort adorably in Jason's ear, then sneezed all over his face. Jason giggled and cuddled the puppy closer. Even I kissed the puppy on his snorting, snoring, sneezing, snorgling, beastly nose. Well, I mean, all that sneezing was just too cute. I admit it. Once again, I was a goner from the get-go. I have zero resistance when it comes to puppies.

So of course, we filled out all the papers, and handed over the adoption fee without an argument, and signed on the dotted line, and accessorized to the hilt. On the next page is just a partial list of what you'll need to bring home a puppy, according to Jason.

So we wrapped the puppy up in his overpriced sweater, bundled him into a cab, and headed for home. Jason could hardly contain his joy. He finally had the pug puppy he'd been dreaming about for years, and I saw a look of excitement in his eyes like I hadn't seen in quite some time. Or maybe ever. And that includes during the Barneys warehouse sale, which is saying something.

Jason named him Elvis right there on the spot. The handle fit. And as I watched Elvis curled up in Jason's lap on his way to his new home, I knew that Elvis was where he belonged, and so, at least for the

PupWallet
Puppy Accessory List

LOTS of wee-wee pads: Because it takes a lot of pads to train a puppy. There are lots of brands on the market now, so find the one that works for you.

Training treats: Ideally, you will want to be training your puppy, so healthy training treats that are especially made for puppies are a must. And until they are ready to train, they'll do really cute stuff just to get a treat.

Vitamin supplement: Just in case your puppy needs a little help growing and flourishing, or is a picky eater, it's good to have a supplement around to help your puppy build strong bones twelve ways.

Puppy clothes: A cute sweater and a cute T-shirt with a bad puppy pun on it, like Barkeologist, and a funny hat aren't absolutely essential, but trust us, they will be lots of fun in the puppy pictures.

Puppy food: Generally, they recommend buying a little of the food that the puppy is currently eating when you take him home. But you will probably want to switch him off the institutional cheap stuff as quickly as you can, so buy the brand you want to switch to, as well. We like Wellness, Triumph, and California Natural, because they are healthy foods with very few by-products, but there are lots of good brands out there to choose from these days. And one word to the wise: while they are growing, puppies tend to eat *a lot*.

(Continued)

A prince or princess bed: Just like everybody, a puppy needs a bed he can call his very own. There are lots of beds to choose from; we like the Bessie & Barnie Bagel Bed, because you can customize the fabric and the cover is removable. But there are lots of great styles to choose from. We suggest natural fibers that are cuddly and *washable!*

Play toys: Introduce play toys early; it keeps puppies from being bored, and they look really cute sleeping on their toy. Great photo ops. We've got a toy chest bigger than a steamer trunk around here. We like the talking toys, like the wise guy that says "Hey, you think I'm funny, what am I a clown?" There are also toys that quack or oink or moo. Toys are as fun for you as for the puppy, so knock yourself out!

Teething toys: Better face it early on: puppies *love* to chew. On *everything.* So give your furniture, your friends, and your fingers a break and buy them some good chew toys for those irrepressible teething urges. We like Merrick's Flossies or bully sticks or Dingo Bones or Nylabones. But experiment with your puppy and find out what he loves to gnaw on best, then stock up!

Harness and leash: You'll need to start leash-training your puppy right away in anticipation of your long walks together. For puppies and dogs, we prefer a harness to a collar, as it doesn't choke the dog and doesn't pull off when he tugs against the lead. There are lots of great brands and styles. Our favorites are Bessie & Barnie Harnesses. They make really cute matching leashes, too.

(Continued)

Baby wipes: Trust me, you'll need moist wipes for *lots* of reasons when you first get a puppy. We don't bother with the ones especially made for pets; we buy baby wipes, preferably with aloe for wiping up the puppy, and with disinfectant for wiping up puppy messes.

Nature's Miracle: This miracle solvent will remove your pet's scent wherever the puppy's had an accident, which is important for pad training. We buy this stuff by the gallon, but they also make it in a spray pump, and pre-moistened wipes, which are a little pricey but very handy.

Baby blanket: Have a soft, cuddly designated blanket that your puppy can cuddle up with on the couch, in the bed, and in the carrier. In times of stress, security blankets work for puppies, too!

Pooch pouch: There are lots of adorable ways to cuddle and carry your new puppy. There are pooch pouches, puppy purses, puppy Björns, marsupial sacks, and slings. Try some on for size and find the best fit for you and your puppy.

moment, were we. I really didn't feel the need to think much further forward than the next block ahead. I didn't see the point; why question anything when everything felt so perfect? We would deal with whatever came, just like we always had. The road ahead looked bright.

And then we got home and came face-to-face with Daisy, and I realized that we had some explaining to do.

Daisy was *not* having it. She took one look at Elvis, whom, incidentally, Jason had dressed in a soft camel sweater with an orange star on the back, which was not helping matters any, and disappeared into her princess bed under the coffee table. Gone was Daisy's canine serenity, gone her Mona Lisa smile, gone her unspoken welcome to whatever was to come. Gone, and replaced by one major Chihuahua 'tude that did not let up for the better part of three weeks. And trust me, when it comes to 'tudes, Chihuahuas are professionals.

I tried to ignore Daisy's unwelcoming attitude, figuring it takes all animals a few days to get used to things. Animals generally work out relations much better than people. And ours was a household based on a harmonious melding of opposites. So I remained optimistic.

"I know what will make everybody feel better," I said one day hopefully. "We'll give Elvis a welcome home party, and I'll make some Welcome Home Elvis Pupcakes. Daisy can eat one, too." When it came to people or puppies, food was always my first and best solution to any dilemma. Daisy looked at me, intrigued, and cocked her head. Well, I had said the "E" word. Here was my calorie prescription. Give this recipe a shot when

Bev's Culinarytherapy

Welcome Home Elvis Pupcakes

Preheat oven to 350 degrees F.

HERE'S WHAT YOU'LL NEED:
1 ripe banana, mashed
1 medium-sized carrot, grated
1 medium-sized zucchini, grated
2 eggs
1/4 cup honey
1/4 cup maple syrup
2 1/2 cups whole wheat flour
1/2 teaspoon cinnamon
1/2 teaspoon nutmeg
1 teaspoon baking powder
Dash salt
4 ounces cream cheese, softened

HERE'S HOW YOU DO IT: Grease and flour a 12-cup muffin pan. Mix together the banana, carrot, zucchini, eggs, honey, and syrup. In another bowl, combine the dry ingredients, then fold into the wet mixture. Add a little water if the mixture is too thick. Scoop with an ice cream scoop into the muffin pans and bake about 45 minutes. Top with cream cheese sweetened with a little honey. Cool before serving to your puppy.

you're trying to grease the wheels. Or, rather, frost them.

While I whipped up the Pupcakes, Jason held Elvis in his lap and stroked his velvety head. He really was just about the cutest puppy I had ever seen. And Jason wasn't exactly tough on the eyes, either.

They were adorable together, and I smiled as I stirred, shaking my head and wondering how I had found myself surrounded by so much cuteness. Daisy glowered at us through the whole Hallmark moment. Even letting her lick the frosting off the spatula didn't cheer her up.

When the Pupcakes were done, Elvis gobbled his greedily and got cream cheese frosting on the top of his nose, then spent the next forty-five minutes trying unsuccessfully to lick it off. Daisy nibbled a few crumbs and then climbed back into her bed, unmoved.

Day in and day out Daisy ignored us, only occasionally acknowledging us with a withering glance from beneath the fluff of her lair. There was no question about it. She was really pissed. And I don't mean just metaphorically pissed; I mean intentionally not peeing on the pad pissed, which was really getting old.

There was one interesting development, however. Nick the cat and Daisy, who had been adversaries, or at best reluctant housemates, suddenly became thick as thieves. They started playing together in the mornings, rolling around on the floor together like they were the two puppies, and completely ignored poor Elvis, who wanted nothing more than to join in the fun. I think that it pretty much sucked to be Elvis at that point. And our laundry bills were through the roof.

Jason and I were beside ourselves. All kinds of circular obsessive thoughts were running through our heads. What if they never made peace? What if they couldn't live together? They were very different dogs, after all. Daisy was smart, Elvis wasn't. Elvis was purebred elegance, Daisy was ghetto fabulous. Elvis was Westminster supermodel gorgeous, and Daisy was, well . . . beautiful in her own nontraditional way. They were a couple that just didn't make sense on the face of things, much like Jason and me. Only whereas Jason and I seemed drawn together by a magnetic force far more powerful than ourselves, Elvis and Daisy were equally repelled.

And there were other issues at play besides pure magnetism. As things stood then, Elvis was Jason's dog and Daisy was mine. So even if Elvis and Daisy found a way to be friends, what would happen when Jason and Elvis moved out? I mean look at us. How would you divide up this picture?

No. Getting another dog hadn't made things easier at all. It had only complicated things. But what were we supposed to do? He was just too cute.

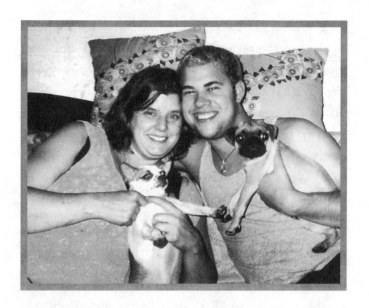

And apparently, we were on a path for a reason, and were destined to stay on it, even though we didn't have the slightest idea where it was leading, or where we would end up.

So, for these reasons and many others that I haven't gotten to yet in therapy, we tried not to think too much about the future. For one thing, with regard to Jason and me and Elvis and Daisy as a family, there technically wasn't a future. There was only a now. It was one of those times when you are forced to live in the present, because the present is all you have.

At times like these, sometimes miracles happen.

But in the meantime, we had to make our own magic, and figure out a way to keep Daisy from biting Elvis's snorting, sneezing, snorgelling pug nose off. We started out with diplomacy. We drew some healthy boundaries and established a designated and well-defined territory for Elvis. It wasn't all that easy to find a designated territory for Elvis in the middle of our already farcically over-burdened junior one-bedroom . . . Which is how Elvis wound up gated in the foyer. This, of course, caused us an enormous amount of guilt, not to mention making it very difficult to go in or out the front door. Elvis would look at us pathetically from behind his healthy boundary, and wag his tail, just waiting for somebody to cross the line, which I did so often in the beginning it was hardly worth defining the boundary at all.

Jason would get firm with me then, and remind me that consistency is key when it comes to any plan with an animal, but then Elvis and I would look up at him, and his resolve would melt. The boundary method was hard on us all, all of us, that is, except for Daisy, who looked relieved with all of Elvis's competing cuteness safely behind bars. Even Nick looked a little guilty, and he was a true cynic when it came to puppies and, well, just about everything. But the gated-room method did turn out to be a very good method for pad-training a puppy, which we discovered, quite by accident.

Daisy did begin to ease up on the attitude a little bit with Elvis safely behind bars. And she started using the pad again, which was a great relief to us all. But there was no doubt about it. She despised Elvis. I tried to confront the sibling rivalry head-on, and reassure Daisy that she was still my baby by putting her in her cashmere puppy sling while I cooked. I'd talk to her while I tried out recipes for a Make the Peace chapter I was fooling around with. I'd give Daisy little nibbles of Gruyère while developing my recipe for Going the Extra Mile Gratin, which by the way can melt any cold war. The recipe is on page 53, for the next time you're trying to help somebody meet you halfway.

Still, despite all our efforts in the kitchen and out, Daisy just wouldn't warm up to Elvis. And while Elvis was a very good sport about things and never seemed to hold a grudge, you could tell that he was getting his feelings hurt. None of us was a very happy puppy. Something had to give.

"Maybe it's hopeless," I said to Jason one day.

Housebreaking for Homebodies

When your puppy is old enough to make choices about where he or she "goes," isolate an area and cover the entire space with pads. This way, the puppy will have no choice but to use the pads every single time he has to go. Praise your puppy whenever he goes on the pad. And as the puppy has no choice, you never have to scold the puppy at the outset. Which is a plus for us softies, believe me. Then, gradually start to take away the pads, while still keeping the puppy in the confined area. Keep a watchful eye on your puppy, and whenever he is looking like it's that time, put the puppy on the pad. At this point puppies will have an option to make a mistake, so you're going to have to find a way to scold that adorable puppy when he goes anywhere *but* on the pad. But only scold the puppy if you catch him in the moment. Dogs don't understand about holding a grudge. When your puppy is getting the hang of things, and going with regularity to the pad, you can eliminate the gate, but leave the pad in the same place. Then, once the puppy is flawless, you can move the pad to a location where you want to keep it permanently and help him to find it. You may have to pay more attention for a few days until the puppy figures out the new pad placement. Using this method, we, who were very stupid humans when it came to dogs in the beginning, were able to pad-train our puppies in about one week.

"Maybe it's like milk and lemons. They don't mix—they curdle."

"WWTFBD?" said Jason. "What would Tammy

Going the Extra Mile Gratin

HERE'S WHAT YOU'LL NEED:

2 Idaho potatoes

2 medium zucchinis

1 large Vidalia onion, cut into halves

3/4 stick unsalted butter

Salt and freshly ground pepper to taste

1 teaspoon fresh thyme leaves

1/4 teaspoon fresh ground nutmeg

3 tablespoons flour

1 cup milk, heated

1 cup Gruyère cheese, grated

1/2 cup bread crumbs

HERE'S HOW YOU DO IT: Pick potatoes and zucchinis that are roughly the same size around so that they cook at the same speed. Slice them both into 1/2-inch rounds. Slice the onion into 1/2-inch rounds. Melt the butter in a cast-iron Dutch oven and add onions, salt, and pepper. Sauté slowly until they are soft, pliable, and semi-caramelized. Go the extra mile and don't rush the onion process. The small amount of extra time you take with this detail at the beginning makes a *huge* difference down the line. Next, toss in zucchinis and potatoes, and a little more salt and pepper, along with thyme and nutmeg, and sauté this mixture for about 5 minutes, until the vegetables are beginning to soften. Then stir in flour, add your milk, and stir until the mixture thickens slightly. Take off the heat, stir in half the cheese, and pour into a 12-inch greased shallow baking dish. Toss the remaining cheese with the bread crumbs and spread over the top. Dot with butter and bake until brown and bubbly and ready to inspire you for the extra mile, but only after having the second helping.

Faye Bakker do? Come on Bev, when life gives you lemons . . ."

"You can't make lemonade out of lemons and curdled milk," I said gloomily.

"No," said Jason, and the sun came out from behind the clouds as he smiled, "but you can make ricotta cheese."

"Wise guy," I said, but truth be told, I was impressed. Because he was right, you know. You can make a fantastic ricotta cheese out of curdled milk and lemons. He'd been listening to me. Here's how you do it, by the way (see next page); it's a little kitchen magic that's really easy and completely satisfying in an instant-gratification sort of way. And there is something fundamentally reassuring about being able to make your own cheese.

"They'll work it out," said Jason, who in his brief twenty-three years had already survived a catastrophic flood that wiped out his town *and* the attack on the World Trade Center, and yet still, fantastically, maintained a healthy faith in the unknown. "If Daisy's mad, then she'll just have to get glad again."

I was skeptical about that. I had seen that look in Daisy's eye. It didn't look like flexibility to me.

"I don't know," I said, moving toward the snarls

When Life Gives You Lemons, Make Ricotta Cheese

HERE'S WHAT YOU'LL NEED:
3 cups milk
Juice of 1 lemon

HERE'S HOW YOU DO IT: Bring 3 cups of milk to a boil, add the juice of 1 lemon, reduce heat, and stir until the milk completely curdles. Next, line a strainer with cheesecloth and place over a large bowl. Pour the curdles through the strainer into the bowl, and allow to drain for a couple of hours. The longer you drain and dry the ricotta, the firmer it will become. When you have reached the consistency you would like, pour into a bowl and refrigerate. Serve this as an appetizer with crackers, and watch how impressed people are when you tell them it's homemade ricotta. You can also stir in a little lemon zest, or sun-dried tomatoes, or just a little salt and pepper. Fresh thyme is quite good also, or parsley or pepperoncini. Get creative and try out some different flavors; ricotta makes a perfect neutral canvas, so don't be afraid to get cheesy with it!

I had just heard coming from the general direction of the bedroom. "I mean, what if Daisy just refuses to accept him? We can't live like this forever."

Neither one of us said it, but we both knew in that moment that there was another choice. Jason and Elvis could move out. This arrangement wasn't designed to be permanent anyway. It was always assumed Jason would find his own place one of these days. We knew that at some point this chapter would end. Maybe Elvis was the final plot point in this episode.

I looked at Jason and knew that this idea had entered his mind, too, and then we both looked at Daisy, who seemed to be considering her options, as well. And then, as usually happens at terrifying moments like this when the possibility of sudden change looms right in front of you before you're ready, we all got very, very hungry.

"Well," I said, doing my very best Scarlett O'Hara, which wasn't that good, to be honest, "I don't want to think about this now, I can't think about it now or I'll go mad. I'll think about it to-morrow. Now let's eat."

I made personal meat loaves. It was one of my tried-and-true recipes for making the peace. It was a particularly effective dish because it was a comfort food with clean boundaries. And best of all, nobody had to share. Personal meat loaves had brokered many a truce during the hostile family take-overs in my background.

So I whipped up two meat loaves for Jason and me and two smaller ones for Elvis and Daisy. I put their plates on opposite sides of the kitchen. Elvis downed his meat loaf in about twelve seconds flat. Daisy nibbled at her meat loaf delicately, giving Elvis the side eye the entire time. When Elvis was done, he bounced in his usual feckless fashion over to Daisy's plate. Daisy began to snarl and bared her teeth, and I moved in to prevent the inevitable carnage, but Jason said, "Wait," and put his arm out, stopping me before I could swoop in and rescue Elvis.

"But she'll take his face off," I said, seriously worried.

"Let's just see what happens," Jason said, and held my hand tight. I have to admit, I was nervous. I'd seen a lot of one-eyed pugs. And this was against everything they had said to do in the puppy books. Every one of them said explicitly that you should separate dogs when they eat, and that's even with dogs that liked each other. Daisy couldn't stand Elvis, and what's more, I knew from experience that she took the personal part of the personal meat loaf *very* seriously.

Elvis bounded up to Daisy in his usual clumsy frat boy way and Daisy snapped at him, nipping him on the nose. Elvis stopped in his tracks, looking stupefied. It was like those cartoon dogs whose eyes pop out of their head, roll around a few times, and then resettle with a ring of stars circling over their head. Elvis is a very Looney Tunes–style creature.

Recovering himself, Elvis lay down facing Daisy and put his chin on his paws. Then, in a final and I might say brilliantly strategic move, given the gray matter he was working with, Elvis began to whimper softly. Jason held my arm tighter. He was going to let this moment play out once and for all. He was tired of being afraid of what might happen. Apparently, so was Elvis.

So Elvis just lay there, dangerously close to Daisy, without moving, staring hungrily at her meat loaf and whimpering at strategic intervals for what seemed like forever. Apparently Elvis was waiting, just like the rest of us, for the inevitable to happen.

Daisy stopped eating and stared at Elvis, focusing every scintilla of her generations-in-the-barrio-bred Chihuahua intensity on the puglet lying just inches from her personal meat loaf. I tensed, waiting for Daisy to pounce. Jason and Nick both were holding their breath . . .

And then, a miracle happened. Daisy left her meat loaf (which was a miracle in and of itself) and walked around behind Elvis. Elvis, sensing that his hour might be near, moved in for his last meal, and kind of wiggled up to the plate on his belly and began to lick at the edges of Daisy's meat loaf. None of us said a word. This was it. Here was the showdown we had been erecting puppy gates to avoid all summer.

Daisy put her nose out, tentatively sniffing Elvis's head, and then, after a teeth-rattling pause, as if considering the implications of her next move carefully, Daisy began to lick the pug's ears while allowing him to eat her entire meat loaf.

The next thing we knew, Elvis and Daisy were chasing each other around the house, rolling around the floor together, transforming themselves into a whirling puppy pile of joy, as if they'd been best friends all their lives. I had to give Jason credit; he had been engineering this moment for a very long time, and it had worked. And so had my meat loaf.

"Chalk up another victory for personal meat loaves," I said, hugging Jason, as Elvis and Daisy went barreling past us and slammed into the couch. And then we started to laugh, both relieved that, for the moment anyway, the chapter of our lives together was still being written.

By the way, our recipe for brokering the peace between warring factions can be found on the next page.

As that first fall unfolded, and we entered the season of crisp and clear blue-sky mornings, Elvis

Personal Meat Loaves for Puppies with Attitude Sauce

(Serves 2 people and 2 puppies)
Preheat oven to 325 degrees F.

HERE'S WHAT YOU'LL NEED:
1 medium-sized yellow onion, minced
2 tablespoons extra virgin olive oil
1 clove garlic, minced
2 pounds ground turkey
1 extra large egg
3 teaspoons salt
1 teaspoon freshly ground pepper
1 teaspoon dried oregano
1/4 cup grated Parmesan cheese
1 cup fresh bread crumbs
Dash Worcestershire sauce
1/2 cup crushed ice

FOR THE ATTITUDE SAUCE:
1/2 cup ketchup
3 tablespoons brown sugar
1/2 teaspoon celery seed
Dash mustard

HERE'S HOW YOU DO IT: Sauté onions in olive oil until caramelized, add garlic, and remove from heat. Set aside to simmer down and cool off. In a large separate bowl, put your meat and all other ingredients except the ice and mix with a fork. Don't overmix—it suffocates all the ingredients and results in a heavy loaf. Finally, add the cooled onion mixture, and toss

(Continued)

with the crushed ice. Form into two small and two large personal meat loaves and place on a pan. Next, with a whisk, whip the ketchup, brown sugar, celery seed, and dash of mustard until glossy. Spread over the top of the loaves and bake at 325 degrees F for 1 hour until loaves are firm and done. Serve separately and with a full loaf length in between diners.

and Daisy's comfortable friendship began to take an unexpected twist.

In the beginning it was subtle. Just a little spark in Elvis's eye now and again, and his becoming completely devoted, like he was a member of the Daisy cult and was fascinated with every minute detail of her daily routine. He spent most of his days looking at Daisy like this.

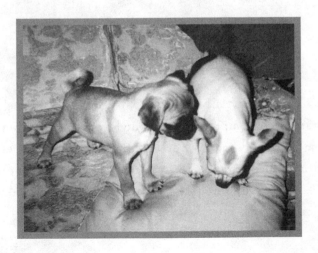

After a time, as Elvis got a little older, we'd find him cuddling up with Daisy on the couch, squeezing as much of his pug puppy body next to Daisy as Daisy would allow. We could tell Daisy was loving the attention, but she managed to maintain a quiet remove. Apparently, she had learned a few things from Nick, as you can see.

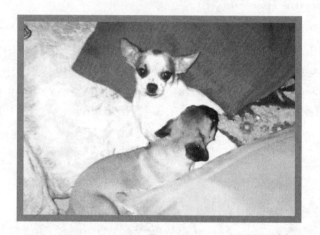

Eventually, Elvis wore Daisy down, and we'd start to come upon them in the love seat, with their paws around each other's necks, doing this unsettling half-biting, half-kissing thing (see next page).

We couldn't help but get the idea that their relationship was becoming something more than in-

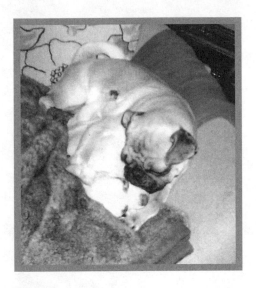

nocent young puppy love. In fact, it looked a lot like heavy petting. Jason and I were appalled.

It's kind of a weird feeling watching your puppies make out on your couch. They'd do it for hours and coo at each other the whole time, and we didn't really understand what it meant. But we knew it was better than growling and snarling, and Elvis was just a puppy, and Daisy wasn't in heat, so we just kind of got used to things and it became just one more thing about our lives that we didn't quite understand. Until one day, the meaning of it all suddenly became clear.

Five

Life Is What Happens While You Aren't Paying Attention

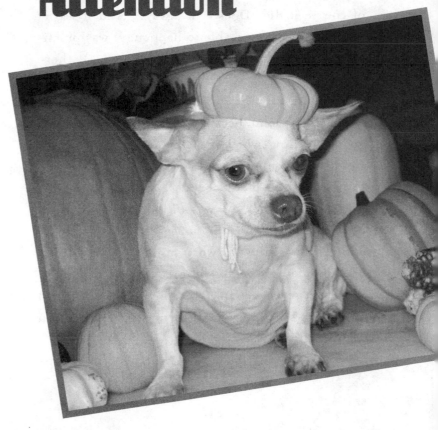

It happened when I wasn't looking. Well . . . of course it did. Doesn't it always? And it wasn't even supposed to be able to happen. It was practically a medical impossibility. And yet . . . there it was.

I was putting the finishing touches on the day's test-kitchen menu, because after all, it was Thanksgiving morning, which is a test cook's dream holiday. Nobody imposes dietary restrictions on Thanksgiving. It was like a blank check.

And Thanksgiving was a high holiday for special reasons around our house because it was the anniversary of the day when Jason and I first met. This should have been a tip-off even way back then. We weren't even a couple, and yet we had celebrated an anniversary every year. I guess sometimes you really are the last person to know.

I was working out a recipe for Grateful Grape

Focaccio, which I knew was one of Jason's favorites. I made it with my own starter, made with Jason's favorite raspberries, and everything I make with it is delicious. Making your own starter is a mystical experience, because you actually create a living organism that can outlive you by hundreds of years. It's a little piece of immortality in a jar. Just think of it: the yeast you make today could be in loaves that are baked by your great-grandchildren. I love that idea.

Anyway, such were my thoughts as I peacefully typed away toward my deadline that morning, when suddenly, I heard a staccato scuffling of paws erupt in the distance. Now, I'm not unaccustomed to that sound. It happens all the time around this joint, so I wasn't immediately clued in to the fact that anything in particular was going on behind my back. But instead of dying down and ultimately collapsing in a cuddly quiet heap of cooing and kissing like usual, this was beginning to escalate into what sounded like a full-fledged doggie smack-down.

Finally I turned around to see what the fuss was all about only to discover that Elvis and Daisy were stuck together. This is a polite way of saying that our big dumb lug of a pug, who was only eight months old and whose left ball hadn't even dropped yet, was nailing our teeny tiny teacup Chihuahua like it was his job.

"Jason!" I screamed. Jason came stumbling out of the bedroom in his underwear looking more than somewhat dazed and looked at me sleepily after hissing twice at the Thanksgiving morning sunshine flooding in through the potted mum and mixed-gourd harvest display we'd carefully arranged the night before. It was havoc with a bucolic backdrop. I pointed at our puppies, practically speechless.

"Elvis . . . Daisy." I couldn't even manage verbs by that point. Jason took one look; his sleepy slits became wide eyes full of sudden realization. Jason sprang into action and grabbed Elvis, who was turned around backward and whimpering pathetically, for obvious reasons. Daisy, on the other hand, was doing the canine equivalent of lighting a cigarette and rolling her eyes. You could almost see the word *amateur* in a bubble above her head. I rushed for the phone to get a hold of the vet, which wasn't going to be easy on Thanksgiving morning.

"My pug is stuck in my Chihuahua," I said breathlessly to the bored vet tech who answered the emergency line that day. It was only eight a.m. and she was already so over it.

"Oh, I'm very sorry to hear that," she said,

which I could tell she wasn't, but regardless wasn't comforting in the least.

"Yes," I said desperately, "I'm sorry too, especially since now he won't come out."

"Well," said the vet tech, totally unimpressed, "there's a bone in the male penis . . ."

"Okay," I said stopping her up short. I really didn't want to search any further in that help index. "Just tell me, how do I get them unstuck?"

"You could try cold water, or KY jelly. Or you can just wait twenty minutes," she said laconically. I swear she was doing her nails while she was talking to me.

And so, for the next twenty minutes, Jason and I sat on the floor looking at each other incredulously and trying to stay calm. We knew something major was happening in that breathless way that you do before you really realize what is coming down the pike at you. Jason held Daisy and whispered in her ear to keep her distracted, while I tried to hold on to Elvis, who was squirming and whining the whole time. We tried cold water, too, but it only made Elvis more upset. And reaching for the lube was further than we were willing to go. So we just waited, and learned that whether you are a person or a puppy, when you come face-to-face with one of the laws of physics, you just have to step back and admit that you can't push, or in this case, pull a river.

And so we waited together for whatever was going to happen next. And finally, after what seemed like about a week and a half, Elvis slipped free, and Jason and I took our first deep breath and collapsed into a cooing, kissing heap with the puppies, laughing with relief that we had once again made it out of

WalletPup
Stress Management Tools for Pups on the Verge

KONGs: They may look like just hollow rubber balls made by the Michelin Man, but put a little peanut butter or cream cheese inside, and a Kong will keep your puppy contented and calm for hours.

Plush talking toys: Elvis will sit and push on his talking toys all day long. He even sleeps with them. And the best part is that he looks amazed every time the toy talks to him. We wish we could be that easily amused! He even does that adorable head-tilt thing sometimes. It's priceless and keeps his pug tail out of trouble for hours. Our favorites are the laughing koala bear and the pig (from Multipet), and we love the rappin' Beef Street Boyz (from Ethical Pet Products).

(Continued)

Kitty Hoots Political Animals: Get your dog interested in politics with these highly partisan doggy hoots from Fat Cat, Inc. They make dolls for folks on both sides of the aisle, which are tough and resilient, and almost never tear when chewed on—although they do come with a squeaker, which Elvis loves and we try to ignore.

Nylabones: Will satisfy even the most orally fixated pup for hours, and have the added benefit of cleaning his teeth.

FURminator deShedding Tool for pets: Nothing calms a dog down like a good brushing, and this amazing new invention easily removes the undercoat. Elvis looked pounds lighter after his first FURmination. And when he's less itchy, he's much easier to get along with.

Salmon or Fish Oil with Omega-3 and -6: Add a little fish oil to your pup's diet. It not only makes for a wonderful coat, boosts immune response, and fights allergies, but has an antidepressant quality that will calm your pet down and brighten his outlook, because, after all, it is a dog's life.

a very tight squeeze, unscathed. Or so we thought at the time.

But something must have told us that we weren't out of the woods yet, because first thing on Friday morning, we made an appointment to have Elvis neutered.

Finally, Thanksgiving evening was upon us. The pilgrims sat down with the Indians, and Elvis

Bev's Culinarytherapy

Here is the recipe for one of my favorite rustic breads and my now famous sourdough starter, at least 'round these parts. The next time you are throwing a feast of thanks, serve this bread hot out of the oven with a stinky triple-cream cheese like La Tur or Robiola, maybe a little raw honey and prosciutto wrapped around some ripe fruit, and a glass of Jason's Harvest Sangria, and I guarantee you will be living from a place of gratitude.

Grateful Grape Focaccia

HERE'S WHAT YOU'LL NEED:
3 1/2 cups flour
3/4 cup cool water
3 tablespoons olive oil
2 teaspoons salt
2 tablespoons honey
3/4 cup sourdough starter (substitute 1
    packet or cake commercial yeast and
    3/4 cup water if you don't want to
    bother with making starter)
Red grapes
Fresh rosemary
Grated Grana Padano
Salt and pepper

HERE'S HOW YOU DO IT: Put the flour in your food processor and take a moment to be grateful that you are not making focaccia by hand. If you have a dough button on your machine, push it. If not, don't worry about it; I'm not entirely sure what it does anyway. Next, put the water, oil, salt, and honey in a measuring cup and whisk together gently. If you are using yeast, dissolve it in a separate cup with 3/4 cup cool water. Turn your machine on, and slowly pour in the starter or yeast mixture through the feeder tube.

(Continued)

Next add the oil, water, and honey mixture and blend until the dough forms a ball. If a ball doesn't form, add more water gradually until it does. Once the ball has formed, say thank you to the gods of the cooking cosmos because dough can be fickle, then let it go around just for good measure. Power down and dump the dough onto a floured board or countertop. Sprinkle some more flour on top, then set it in an oiled bowl to rise (about 1 hour) until doubled in bulk. Yeast is such a gratifying medium. I love when things double in bulk. Once the dough has doubled, pour it out onto the board again, stretch it out a little, and shape it into a free-form, organic expression of your current state of mind. Push your fingertips into the dough to make little indentations all over the focaccia. Artfully press in some grapes, fresh rosemary sprigs, sprinkle with Grana Padano, salt, and pepper. You can get creative, too—throw on a little goat cheese, a little fresh oregano. This is one of those recipes designed to let you use whatever you've got lying around the house. Let the loaf rise for another 30 to 45 minutes, until the loaf gets all puffed up and fluffy, then bake at 450 degrees F (preferably on a bread stone in the bottom of your oven) for about an hour.

Bev's Famous Sourdough Starter

A good active starter takes about 7 to 10 days to produce. But it will live forever!

HERE'S WHAT YOU'LL NEED:
1/2 pint red raspberries
3 cups white flour
2 cups water

HERE'S HOW YOU DO IT: Gently wash the raspberries and tie them into a bundle in cheesecloth. In a large glass container, make a slurry of the flour and water, and submerge the bundle in the slurry. Cover and allow to stand for a couple of days. On the third day, add another cup or 2 of flour

(Continued)

and about 1/2 cup of water, stir, replace the cover, and then feed with flour and water daily until the starter is bubbling and smooth and milky. After about 7 to 10 days, your starter should be active enough to make dough rise, so whip up a batch of grape focaccia, then stand back and watch history in the baking!

Jason's Barmacy

Harvest Sangria

When the leaves start to change and the nights cool down, make a batch of this harvest sangria and celebrate the seasons.

HERE'S WHAT YOU'LL NEED:
1 bottle dry red wine
1/2 cup Grand Marnier or Cognac
Juice of 1 orange
1 tablespoon fresh lime juice
1/3 cup superfine sugar
1 pint fresh raspberries
1 apple, peeled, cored, and cut into slices
1/2 lemon, thinly sliced
1/2 orange, thinly sliced
1 pear, cored and cut into chunks
1 bottle raspberry-flavored seltzer water
Ice

HERE'S HOW YOU DO IT: Combine everything but the seltzer water and ice in a large container. Cover and throw it in the fridge for at least 3 to 4 hours (or longer). Before serving, add the seltzer, pour into a tall glass over ice, and enjoy!

sat down *next* to Daisy, as opposed to on top and behind her, and we all broke bread and gave thanks
that we were full, and happy, and together.

Later that night, when everyone had gone home
and we were finally cuddled up in front of the fireplace watching *It's a Wonderful Life* for the forty-fourth
time, Jason and I raised our Macy's Floats, and
clinked our glasses, grateful to each other and the
powers that be that we had had the good fortune to
meet each other on that fateful Thanksgiving Day
three years earlier. Just like that Thanksgiving, we
had no idea yet that this Thanksgiving was becoming yet another anniversary of an event that we
would never forget.

Six

Rebuilding Nirvana

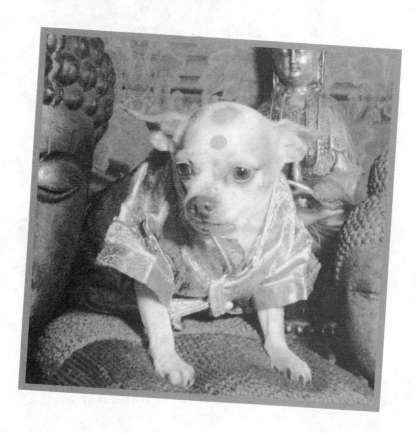

As the holiday season unfolded, we began to realize that our rent-stabilized, parlor-floor brownstone, junior one-bedroom, which had been our haven and our heaven, our shelter from the shit storm of life at the beginning of the twenty-first century, was falling down around our ears.

It's funny how you never realize how important the simple creature comforts are until they go out from under you. And in our case, they didn't go slowly, but as was usually the way with us, they went in the blink of an eye. One day, the radiator in the living room went out and within four hours we could see our breath in the apartment. Next, a pipe burst in the wall and our kitchen flooded. Before we knew it, the landlord had hired a demo crew to gut our kitchen, and then promptly ran out of money. So the workers left, leaving only a shell of a kitchen behind them. And the radiator still didn't work.

And, as it turned out, we still hadn't even come close to hitting bottom.

That winter we had no heat, hot water only intermittently, no kitchen floor, no refrigeration, no kitchen walls, and no extermination. Our stove had been moved out onto the terrace. Mice had moved into the oven. It was like we had been thrust back a hundred and fifty years and found ourselves in the middle of a Charles Dickens novel, with our landlady cast in the role of Scrooge. It was like our junior one-bedroom had become a metaphor for the total disintegration of Western civilization.

Elvis, Daisy, Jason, and I all put on a brave face and made do as best we could. We bought a hot plate and pulled a mattress in front of our fireplace, which, thank God, worked. We rang up a king's ransom in wood deliveries from the local deli and started looking for a lawyer. We fought our way back out of the Dark Ages before plumbing and refrigeration one HPD housing inspector at a time. And gradually, we did make progress. I also became remarkably creative with the hot plate.

We tried to keep our chins up and our toes warm, but one week before Christmas, when they finally took out the living room floor so they could lay a new one sometime the following Wednesday, we buckled. Enough was enough. So we packed our puppies and our flagging Christmas spirits, and headed for the Soho Grand while we waited for our world to change. My agent at the time had suggested the Grand because they accepted dogs. As we discovered, they did a lot more than accept dogs— they pretty much rolled out the puppy red carpet.

When we got to the room, after throwing ourselves into the down softness and heaving a huge and family-wide sigh of relief, we checked out the amenities. The Grand offered puppy canapés, puppy spa treatments, and four-star doggie entrées round the clock. And if you don't have a pet, they'll give you a goldfish, free of charge. Now *that* is what I call pet friendly. You can even bring your dog to happy hour. What temporarily exiled pet owner could ask for anything more? Once we looked into it, we found that there are a lot of places rolling out the puppy red carpet for roving people and their pets these days. Some of our favorites are on the next page.

Fortunately, I had just had a big book check come in, so while it lasted, we threw caution to the wind, bought ourselves matching Chinese pajamas at the Tibetan store, and little matching kimonos for Elvis and Daisy on Canal Street, and moved into a deluxe hotel room in the sky. We shopped,

Petfabulous Palaces for Best Friends on the Fly

The Soho Grand and the Tribeca Grand in New York City offer a full room-service menu for puppies, as well as puppy spa treatments, and will even give you a goldfish if you are missing your own pet.

The Mandarin Oriental in Miami also welcomes puppies, and even provides a doggie welcome kit and a dog bed in every room!

Westin Hotels offer miniature Heavenly Beds brand duvets. Some Westins even offer plush puppy robes, leashes, and collars.

The W Hotels greet every dog with a toy upon check-in, and amenities include in-room puppy massages by a licensed dog massage therapist.

Monaco Hotels maintain an in-house vet, one-hour doggie hikes, and even a video library designed especially for puppies.

Loews Hotels greet every canine guest with a sightseeing map designed especially for dogs. And rooms come complete with toys and treats.

we ate dinner in bed, we slept in sheets that were not covered in plaster dust, we didn't see a single rodent, and it turned out to be the best vacation of our lives, right in our own hometown.

And best of all, Daisy was in heaven. She was

eating like there was no tomorrow, which was her favorite thing in the world, and to be honest, it was beginning to show around her middle. Daisy was developing love handles. And I also began to notice that she wasn't alone. Plus, all that Daisy seemed to want to do in between meals was sleep and cuddle. She had no interest in a puppy massage or a trot on the puppy treadmill at the doggie gym. Yet she didn't seem sick. In fact, if a Chihuahua could be said to have an inner glow, Daisy's dimmer was thrown up to full.

But Jason and I were too busy eating and sleeping and relaxing ourselves for the first time in what seemed like a century to notice. We were basking in our brief respite, and enjoying a little pure, uncomplicated, and vastly overpriced fun together and beginning to understand that necessity was not the only tie that was binding us. We really loved each other and we loved being a family. Which was a good thing, as it turned out, because unbeknownst to us, our family was about to double in size.

The curtains of denial were pulled back by an unseen hand, and the truth of what was happening to us was finally and somewhat embarrassingly revealed the moment we moved back into our court-mandated renovated apartment and our house-warming party guests got a gander at Daisy's belly.

When she was upright, it practically dragged on the floor. We figured it was all that rich room service she'd ordered. And then we hadn't been socializing much since moving back into our freshly ghetto-renovated but now completely empty pad, and we'd been spending a lot of time just us and the dogs, trying to imagine what our new world was going to look like.

We bought a martini bar in Chelsea and designed the whole room around that. And as you can see on the next page, Elvis really got into the Stork Club spirit of things at our new bar.

Don't worry. Elvis didn't inhale. Truth be told, Elvis had been glowing lately, too. In fact, we all were. Things were definitely looking up. But when we finally reopened the doors to Bev and Jason's Bar and Grill, we at last got the dose of reality that we, and Daisy, so desperately needed.

"What's Daisy been up to? She looks preggers," said our drag queen friend Princess, who was known for putting his ring finger right on the horn of a dilemma. Princess tossed back his cocktail imperiously, wolfed down a couple of kip nips, and went to inspect Daisy's girth, then looked her dead in the eye.

"Daisy, have you been catting around?"

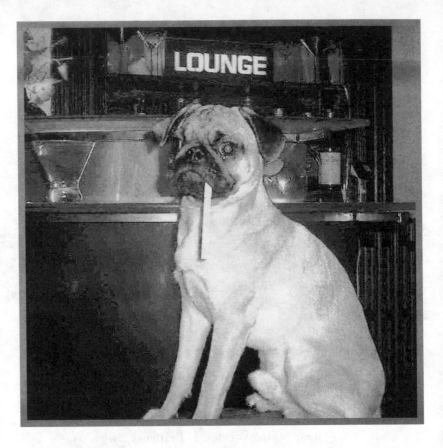

"She's just retaining water," I said.

"Me, too," said Jason, but neither of us sounded very convinced. Although I was trying my hardest to believe myself, something whispered in my ear that I was no longer the sadder but wiser divorcée with the pocket pooch. I had stepped into a new movie. But which one was it?

Two days later found us at the nearest holistic (read "wholly overpriced") veterinary clinic, where I told yet another bored vet tech with an impeccable manicure that I thought our Chihuahua was pregnant. Everyone in the crowded waiting room burst out laughing.

Fourteen hundred dollars and two sonograms later, we knew for sure that Daisy was pregnant, and that she was going to have four puppies, which was a lot for a first birth. Of course Daisy would stretch the seams on that score, too. Further, because a pug's head was so much larger than a Chihuahua's, the vet told us that Daisy was probably going to need a C-section. I started doing the mental calculations and realized that I had better become Mary Higgins Clark, pronto.

Of course, the issue of a puppy abortion did come up. I believed in Daisy's right to reproductive freedom, and if this pregnancy was going to threaten her health, then Daisy's health was going to come first. Remember, though, we were in a holistic Manhattan vet clinic. Nothing is impossible in a place like this. Sure, they had a concern for

Daisy's health. But they also had a first-class birthing specialist, a top-flight surgeon in the event of a C-section, a puppy sonogram machine, and probably even a birthing pool and a breathing class—but I'm not positive about that last part.

"Maybe there is a special pughuahua or chug that needs to be born," said the vet, smiling. Who were we, after all, to deprive destiny of this special puppy, whoever he or she might be? Perhaps this was a puppy that would improve the destiny of dogs everywhere. You just never knew. So we swallowed the pitch line and carried on with the pregnancy and never looked back.

And as the time got closer, Jason and I started to get really excited about the puppies' arrival. Jason had been making accessories lists for weeks, and we were feeding Daisy all kinds of healthy supplements and treating her to the best that puppy holistic health had to offer.

And of course, Jason attended to the style elements of the project. He found four little matching hoodies, all in different colors so we would be able to tell them apart. And he had named each one in advance, which made me nervous. The vet had warned us that it was unusual for all of the puppies to survive in a situation like Daisy's. I was

PupWallet
The Holistic Apawthecary

Derm Caps: This is a concentrated fatty-acid supplement that will give your pet a wonderful shiny coat, and really cuts down on itching and hot spots. It's made with Omega-8 and Omega-3 fatty acids, like safflower oil, borage seed oil, fish oil, and vitamin E.

Super Joint Enhancer: Made by 1-800-PetMeds, this is a great supplement for dogs with arthritis or other joint problems. And just as with people, it actually rebuilds their joint tissue. It comes in liquid, powder, or flavored chewable form, and really helps reduce the tenderness and swelling of arthritis. Chondroitin and glucosamine improve flexibility and mobility, and MSM helps ease pain.

Super VitaChews: Also from 1-800-PetMeds, this is the most complete and healthy multi-vitamin on the market and is loaded with vitamins, minerals, and antioxidants. It has a great anti-aging formula to protect your dog's brain, heart, kidneys, eyes, liver, and immune system. And they taste great!

Nordic Naturals Arctic Cod Liver Oil: This all-natural oil, made from wild Arctic cod, supports healthy cells, skin and coat, joints, heart, brain, eyes, and energy. It's high in vitamin D, which supports healthy vision, bones, and immune function. And it's also great for the digestive system.

worried that naming them would make it that much more difficult if one or two didn't make it.

But Jason said we'd cross that bridge when and if

we got to it, and in the meantime, we might as well plan for the best. So we busied ourselves feathering Daisy's nest and getting ready for the puppies to make their appearance on the scene. Here is our puppy birthing-kit list, half of which we turned out not to need, but we were prepared for every contingency.

Daisy's Birthing Kit

1. Leopard-print Cleopatra tent with plume on top and bean-bag pillow insert
2. 3 fresh, clean, super-absorbent towels
3. A heating pad
4. 2 anti-anxiety pills (for us)
5. Surgical gloves to fill with hot water to keep the puppies warm
6. 4 nursing bottles
7. A cardboard box lined with old pajamas and sheets (once we figured out Daisy wasn't going anywhere near the Cleopatra tent)
8. A collapsible fence
9. A low basket lined with a pillow
10. Puppy formula
11. Nursing vitamin supplements for Daisy
12. Daisy's easy-listening tape, with all the songs that Jason had been singing to the puppies in her belly.
13. 1 large bottle of hydrogen peroxide
14. 1 large bottle of vodka (also for us)

gue shoot. But she
we watched and
oughts, and ex-
Daisy to either
rst. Either one
k a lot of fruit
ame up with.
nexpectedly,
t all along,

ason's pil-

isy to have
or-
go-
turally,
second
order t
ted at the
screen and
y looked like
the tips of our
Maybe Daisy could
the largest puppy, a
tly the same size as
t, of course, recom-
ve had no choice but to
to put Daisy at risk. She
t to help Daisy's chances of
Apparently, Daisy had picked
weight. It was a harbinger of
we didn't know it yet.

aisy home and cut down her por-
e could. She was ravenous and not
he diet. Jason came up with a puppy
nie that she loved, and I tried hard to
o keep her happy while still counting the
We fussed over her regimen like she was a

supermodel getting ready for a *V*
still didn't look any thinner. So
tried to think thin and positive t
ercise discipline, and we waited fo
give birth or pop, whichever came f
looked imminent. And we all dran
smoothies. Below is the recipe Jason c

And then one morning, quite u
even though we had been expecting
Daisy's time finally came.

It was six a.m. Daisy waddled up to J

Jason's Barmacy

Daisy's Suck-It-In Smoothie

HERE'S WHAT YOU'LL NEED:
1 small container plain yogurt (8 ounces)
1/2 cup raspberries
1/2 cup blackberries
1 peach, sliced
1 very ripe banana
1 tablespoon honey
1 cup ice

HERE'S HOW YOU DO IT: For people, blend all the ingredients, th
pour into tall glasses with straw. For puppies, pour into ice cube tra
and freeze, and then serve as a treat after they turn up their snouts at th
steamed rice and vegetables.

low while he was sleeping. She tried to wake him up by licking his face and when that didn't work, she threw up on his pillow. That did the trick. Jason leapt up more quickly than I have ever seen him get out of bed. While he was yelling, "It's time, it's time!," Daisy, listening to a voice far more powerful than our shrill announcements, put her haunches in the air and started to pant. Then Jason started to pant, too, and I realized I had better get this moving quickly before Jason became completely immobilized by sympathy contractions.

We bundled Daisy into her carrier and hailed a cab at rush hour. Somehow we got one right away. The cab goddess was definitely with us and Daisy that morning. She seemed very upset in the cab, with a look in her eye that asked where we were taking her when all she wanted to do was climb into the cardboard box we'd set up for her and give birth quietly at home where she belonged. We rushed into the vet's office and handed her over to the vet tech, who for once looked genuinely concerned.

"That's okay, Mommy," she said, pulling Daisy out of her carrier and putting her over her shoulder. "We're going to take good care of you." Daisy was panting, looking completely unconvinced. And as the vet tech carried Daisy away into the bowels of the procedure room, she kept her startled eyes glued on us, and didn't break contact until the doors of the procedure room shut in her face, and she disappeared from sight. We stood there with tears in our eyes and wondered how we were going to get through the next several hours.

I think that afternoon was one of the longest of our lives. We tried to carry on as usual, but Elvis just lay disconsolately in the foyer, staring at the door, waiting for Daisy's return, which didn't make things any easier. We did what we could to kill the endless time. We ate and we drank and we napped and watched trashy TV. And then we ate and drank again. On the next page is a recipe for Jason's Mellow-Out Mojitos, which really made the seconds fly like hours instead of days.

Finally, after what seemed like a year and a half, the vet's office called at about five o'clock that night. We all held our breath while we waited for her to get on the line. It was, to say the least, a long and pregnant pause. And then, finally, "They're all fine," came the vet's cheerful voice. "We had to work on the two smallest puppies for an hour to get them to breathe, but Mom and all four puppies are doing just fine."

"Thank you so much," I stammered and gave

Jason's Barmacy

Mellow-Out Mojitos

When the heat is on, shake up one of these Mellow-Out Mojitos and
cool out.

HERE'S WHAT YOU'LL NEED:
4 strawberries
1 tablespoon fine sugar
4 basil leaves
2 ounces good rum
Juice of 1 lime
Ice
Seltzer water

HERE'S HOW YOU DO IT: In a tall Old-Fashioned glass, add the (sliced)
strawberries, the sugar, and the basil leaves. Crush and muddle them.
Add the rum, lime juice, and ice. Top off with a splash of seltzer water,
and enjoy!

BARTENDER'S TIP: Excellent Mojitos all have one very important thing
in common: they are made with a muddler. Muddlers are used to bruise
the herbs and fruit, which releases their oils and flavor. They are easy to
find and inexpensive.

Jason the thumbs-up. Jason had been right. We had
expected the best, and the best had happened.

Then the vet said, "You can take them home
tonight."

"Tonight?"

Suddenly time sped up.

Seven

The Puppy
Bowl

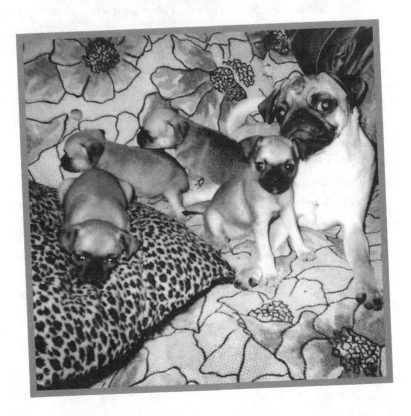

Two rush-hour cab rides and one three-thousand-dollar C-section later, we were on our way home with Daisy and her four new puppies, two boys and two girls, whom Jason had named Buddha, Bert, Betty, and Busta.

We carried Daisy and her puppies home in one of those scary-looking, airline-approved carriers they give you at the vet when you don't have one of your own. They'd tucked the puppies in with surgical gloves filled with hot water. Daisy looked exhausted but happy to be headed home with us, but she didn't look too sure about the puppies who were snuggling up to her belly, which now had thirty-two angry-looking stitches in it because she had not only just had a C-section, but had been simultaneously spayed. No, Daisy didn't look too sure about the puppies at all.

The second we walked through the door, Elvis

was on top of us, trying frantically to climb into the carrier with his new family. We locked him in the bathroom until we got Daisy and the puppies settled. He howled mercilessly from the bathroom and would not be quiet, no matter how many Flossies or Smackos we tossed at him.

We put Daisy and the puppies inside a fenced-off little corner of the living room by the fire. We'd built a bed inside for Daisy, and she settled in gratefully and looked ready to fall into a coma of exhaustion—that is, until we laid the puppies by her. As soon as she sensed one of the puppies, Daisy became immediately stiff, and even snarled a little, which appalled us. What's more, she looked like she seriously might bite the puppy, who was obliviously clawing at her belly in a blind search for a nipple. For real. I thought she was going to bite Buddha's head off.

But true to form, Jason wasn't flapped in the slightest.

"Daisy! Don't be such a crabby bitch," he scolded her. And then more sweetly, "Those are your puppies." Daisy looked at him and seemed to realize on some level that he was right, and that she was being unreasonable. Then Jason picked Daisy up and held her on his lap, and held the puppies up to her belly one by one, and she let them nurse. Gradually, Daisy relaxed, and then Jason laid them all down together in the bed by the fire. Daisy looked up at him with kind of a wistful look in her eyes. To this day, I'm still not sure what she was thinking about or wanted Jason to tell her, but here's the look.

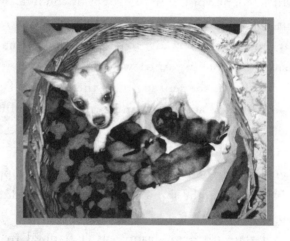

Kind of Mona Lisa–like, don't you think? Daisy always *had* been enigmatic. But Jason understood her immediately, and smiled at her, and kissed her on the head, and five minutes later, they looked like this (see next page).

As usual, our moment of peace was short-lived. Elvis began howling from the bathroom,

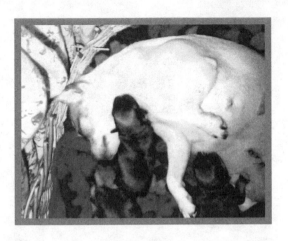

and we finally let him out and waited for all hell to break loose. But instead of charging up to the scene as we'd expected him to, Elvis walked carefully up to the cage and peered politely in at Daisy and the puppies. He didn't start barking and pawing at the fence to knock it down. He didn't rush the gate or make a scene. In fact, he didn't make a move or a sound. He stood, taking a long first look at his new family, and then looked up at us with the same question in his eyes that Daisy had had.

Jason gave Elvis the same answer he'd given Daisy, and patted him on the head, and then Elvis lay down quietly next to Daisy outside the fence and just watched them while they slept.

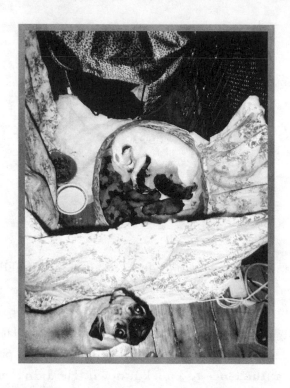

We learned later that when dogs have C-sections, they don't always recognize their puppies as their own because they didn't go through the birth canal. It's very important to get the puppies to nurse, though, because they get important immune-boosters from the mother's milk. So as it turned out, those first moments introducing Daisy to her new litter had been critical, and Jason had stepped in, and in his usual casual and cheerful way, had made all the difference.

And life went on, as it has a tendency to do, but things sure did look and feel a lot different than they had before. Those first weeks with the puppies made me think of something that my friends with babies always used to say to me.

"No matter how hard you think it's going to be," they'd tell me, shaking their heads and smiling like Yoda, "believe me, it's much, much harder." Jason and I were learning the truth of that statement, one bottle feeding at a time.

Some things remained the same. We were still living in my junior one-bedroom—the one that I was worried wouldn't fit one dog, let alone six. And Jason still hadn't thrown out his media collection. But my concerns about storage space had become a small leak in the flood of new parenting responsibilities that now dominated our lives. It took all four of us to care for the new puppies, so it was definitely a time when all hands were needed, whether or not there was room on deck.

It was relatively easy right in the beginning. Before their eyes opened, the puppies were all about Daisy. She was the only thing they could really recognize without eyes, although they got pretty familiar pretty quickly with the tip of the nursing bottle, as well. For me, it was all about keeping Daisy properly nourished. I was throwing calories at her like it was my job. The vet had said she needed twice the calories she normally did, which for a Say-I-Love-You-with-Food chef like me was like a ticket to ride.

I was feeding her peanut butter biscuits and liver pâté, omelets, and fillets. I was tossing her treats whenever she asked for them. Well, we needed to keep Daisy nursing, I'd tell myself. And it was, in my own defense, the truth. Whatever Daisy didn't manage to provide for the puppies, we had to provide, one eye-dropper at a time. And they ate about twelve times a day. Puppies are really hungry creatures, as it turns out. So we learned very quickly that it was in our best interests to keep Daisy well nourished. And after all, we told ourselves, she was eating for five.

Once the puppies' eyes opened and they started to move about the cabin, things got scary. And then, to make matters worse, about six weeks in, it was like an internal alarm clock went off inside Daisy, and she left her nursing basket, climbed back into her princess bed, and began demanding

Yummy Chummies like it was her job. In between naps, that is. Here she is. As you can see, motherhood turned her from Mona Lisa into the Buddha. Bigger belly, happier smile, but still enigmatic.

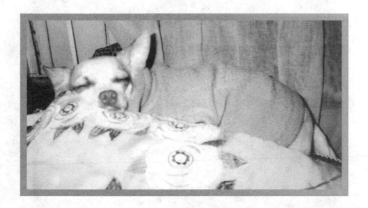

Fortunately, nature abhors a vacuum, and where Daisy left off, Elvis and Jason, the OCD dads, filled in. They hovered over the puppies more than Daisy ever had. Elvis, who was not known for his intellectual prowess, actually learned to count the puppies one by one every time he returned to the basket. And Jason was right behind him, checking the math. I took over the bottle-feeding shifts in the morning, Jason fed them at night, and Elvis spent just about every waking hour cleaning and fussing over his brood until they had to wiggle away from him to keep from getting smothered. No question about it, Elvis was a natural-born psycho dad. Just look at him. He looks so proud. Bewildered, but proud.

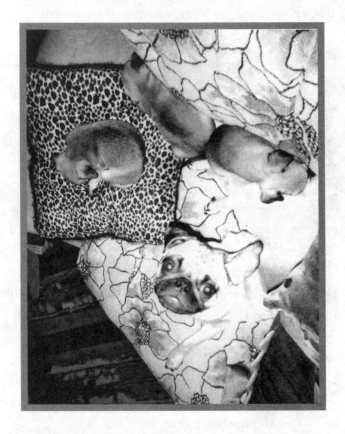

The trouble was, where Daisy had been something of a disciplinarian, and almost a little structured and military in her approach to parenting,

Elvis was scattered and disorganized and distinctly free-form. Elvis did his best, running after each one, frantically trying to keep them all out of harm's way. But the task usually proved to be too much for him. This is when Jason would take over.

They learned to work like a team. Elvis would go rushing off to extricate Bert from some near-disaster, which left Buddha free to wander off and go chew on the nearest power cord. So Jason would go rushing to the rescue, leaving Busta to climb off in yet another direction entirely and do something stupid, like getting caught in the drape. Then Betty

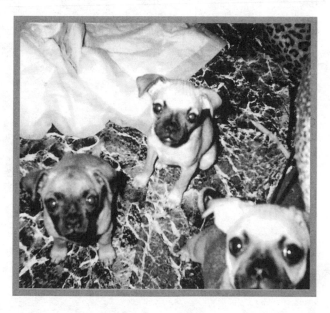

would scream from the bedroom and the whole three-ring puppy circus would begin anew. Well, look at them. Do they just scream out *trouble* or what?

Eventually, when the puppies were finally fed and sleeping in their basket, Elvis would collapse in an exhausted heap next to Daisy and let her clean his ears. Nick watched our antics from his lofty cat perch, far above it all, and was just generally pretty disgusted with us, as usual. Jason would put his head in my lap and I'd stroke his hair, and then all of us would nod off, wondering how in the world we had ever managed without each other.

Life had definitely become a team sport.

Eight

The Language of
Letting Go

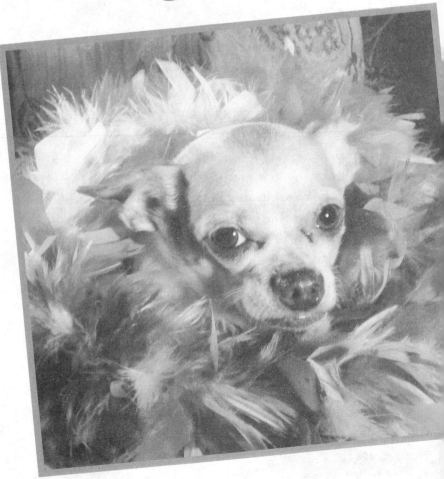

Gradually, the puppies began to look like puppies, and we started to see who they were as individuals.

Buddha was brave and fierce, with short little legs, a velvet apricot coat, and Daisy's determination in her eyes.

Busta was the giant; silent and sweet, with a thick, dark coat dusted with silver and a look of almost saintly endurance. Betty had high spirits, and was always in a fever of excitement, with a zealot's gleam in her eye, and impossibly long legs that were learning very rapidly how to leap tall doggie gates in a single bound. And then there was Bert. Little Bert. The runt of the litter, who had to be coaxed to eat and venture out of the nest, who scratched a lot for no apparent reason, snarled occasionally at Nick, and slept curled up every night with his arm around Daisy's neck. And somehow we had to pick

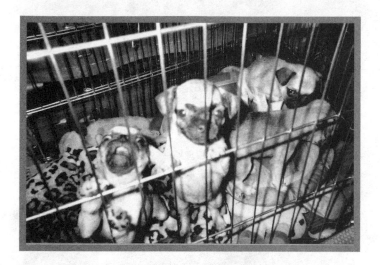

only one puppy to keep. Jason wanted Bert. I wanted Buddha.

The day that Kristen, Busta's new mom, came to pick him up, we were beside ourselves all day long. Jason took a nine-hour nap, Elvis sat on the edge of the couch with his chin on his paws and pouted, and Daisy spent her whole day stress-eating. I was baking stress brownies (see recipe on next page). They work *every* time, no lie.

The brownies helped, but there was still a lump in our throats. And it was more than just dark chocolate. We'd always known this day would come, but now that it was here, we didn't know what to do with ourselves. It was like waiting for the other shoe to drop. We just wanted it to be over already. We all felt dreadful. But when Kristen arrived that night, with a brand new pooch pouch already strapped to her shoulders, and a big shiny smile, you just couldn't help but feel happy for them both.

I guess I should have been wondering at this moment what it was going to feel like when it came

Bev's Culinarytherapy

Stress Brownies

Preheat the oven to 350 degrees F.

HERE'S WHAT YOU'LL NEED:
1 pound unsalted butter
1 pound plus 12 ounces semisweet
    chocolate chips, divided
6 ounces unsweetened chocolate
6 extra-large eggs
3 tablespoons instant coffee granules
2 tablespoons pure vanilla extract
2 1/4 cups sugar
1 cup plus 1/4 cup all-purpose flour, divided
1 tablespoon baking powder
1 teaspoon kosher salt
3/4 cup smooth peanut butter

HERE'S HOW YOU DO IT: Butter and flour a 12 × 18 × 1 1/2-inch sheet pan. Melt together the butter, 1 pound of chocolate chips, and the unsweetened chocolate in a medium bowl over simmering water. Allow

(Continued)

to cool slightly. In a large bowl, stir (do not beat) together the eggs, coffee granules, vanilla, and sugar. Stir the warm chocolate mixture into the egg mixture and allow to cool to room temperature.

In a medium bowl, sift together 1 cup of flour, the baking powder, and the salt. Add to the cooled chocolate mixture. Toss the remaining 12 ounces of chocolate chips in a medium bowl with 1/4 cup of flour, and then add them to the chocolate batter. Pour into the prepared sheet pan. Spoon the peanut butter over the top of the chocolate mixture and, using a knife, swirl it through the chocolate mixture.

Bake for 20 minutes, and then rap the baking sheet against the oven shelf to force the air to escape from between the pan and the brownie dough. Bake for about 10 to 15 minutes more or until a toothpick comes out clean. Do not overbake! Allow to cool thoroughly, refrigerate, and cut into large squares.

time for Jason to leave. But for some reason, I just didn't worry about that anymore. I think we both knew in some unspoken way that neither one of us was going anywhere, even if we weren't able to say it out loud quite yet.

I could tell that Jason was ready to cry as he waved good-bye to Kristen and Busta as they walked down the stairs. When we heard the door finally slam shut downstairs, we burst out into tears, and hugged each other, and felt better. Later that night, Kristen sent us pictures of Busta in his new home. He looked a little confused but happy, and he was surrounded by a mountain of new toys right smack-dab in the middle of Kristen's bed. Her cat looked really pissed.

The next morning, we woke up and immediately set about finding a home for Betty the bouncing chug. We had called everyone we knew, but to be honest we were striking out because Betty was, well . . . bouncing Betty. She hadn't gotten her name by accident. This puppy was bouncing off the walls. She was, as we described it to potential parents, very enthusiastic about life.

Even our vet had returned her. She took her home ostensibly for a trial weekend and brought Betty back the very next morning, saying something about the drapes, and her other dog, who apparently had been terrorized. It wasn't an encouraging sign. Fortunately, fate got creative at just the right moment, and the very same bored vet tech with the impeccable nails who had coached me through the puppies' conception fell in love with our problem puppy, and adopted her on the spot.

When the day came for Betty to go to her new home, I kissed her good-bye with tears in my eyes, and Jason carried her up to the clinic in a backpack. We dressed her in her amber pullover, and sent a carrot that smelled like Daisy along with her to remember us by. I sat quietly with Daisy and the other two puppies until Jason got home. Jason walked through the door and immediately put his head on my shoulder and we both started to cry. We were a very weepy bunch lately. Neither one of us had ever been very good at letting go. But we were learning. Sort of.

And then Jason, quite out of the blue, said, "I want to keep both Bert and Buddha," and looked at me, along with Elvis and Daisy and Bert and Buddha. They all had exactly the same look in their eyes. It said, *Say yes.*

And so I said, "Okay, we'll keep both."

"And I don't want to move out, either," Jason said, also quite out of the blue.

And then I said, "Good, because I don't want you to leave. Ever."

Nine

Pug-
therapy

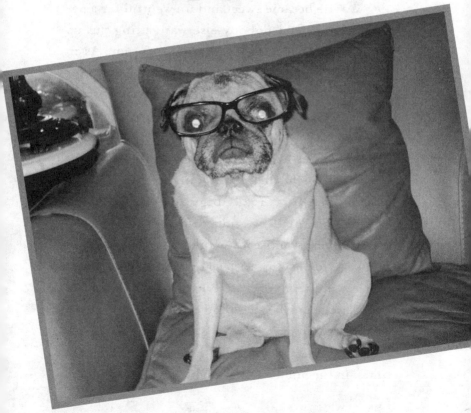

Life became sweet and uneventful for a period. Thank God nobody else was getting put up for adoption, which was a great relief for me. As an adopted child myself, I had an uncontrollable tendency to anthropomorphize when it came to giving puppies away, so I was glad that that part, anyway, was over.

And it was a great relief not to live with the constant thought that I was going to have to let go of a life that I was really beginning to love a lot. It was both a thrilling and a difficult experience to live with no promise of a future, and a constant awareness of having to let go, even of the things that are most important. But for the moment, at least, Jason and I had found the sense of security we had been looking for in each other and in our growing family of dogs. Although I think sometimes, in the middle of the night, we both wondered how long an unlikely union like ours could realistically last.

But in the meantime, our life was going on all around us. The puppies were getting bigger every day, and so, we noticed, was Daisy. I finished my cookbook, which I wrote during what I am sure will be one of the hardest but best periods of my life. When I turned the manuscript in, my editor wrote me a note telling me that when she pulled the manuscript out of the envelope, it smelled like wood smoke. I thought back to that crazy, Grand Guignol Christmas, and wondered how we got through it. Then I remembered. We'd had each other.

With the book finished, and our apartment shining once more like a well-polished, Gilded Age jewel box, and our epic housing-court battle won, and the pets happy, it was time to admit victory and begin a new project. This, for some reason, can be a hard thing for me to do. Well, it's that letting go thing again. Uncertainty and hardship had ironically become familiar friends.

So the summer unfolded while the puppies played, and Daisy ate bonbons, and Nick slept on the radiator growing ever more ancient and disapproving. And then one day, Nick, who had been with me through my wedding, my divorce, my brave new life as a newly single woman in the city, and now my life surrounded by Jason and a lot of dogs, climbed down off of the radiator, snuggled up very close to Daisy, who had always been his favorite, put his head down by hers, and died.

Daisy didn't move from that spot where Nick had lain for a very long time. Even after we'd picked up Nick and carried him to the vet and come home again, Daisy remained in that spot. All through dinner, she wouldn't budge, and late into the night, while we were raising our glass many times to Nick, she just sat quietly in that very same spot. Finally, her appetite got the better of her and we coaxed her into the kitchen for a midnight snack. She ate a little and then went right back to the very same spot and wouldn't even come to bed when we called her.

In the morning, I found her there still, asleep in the first shafts of sunlight coming through the window, on the first morning in many, many years when Nick was not demanding tuna the second I got out of bed. I sat down next to Daisy and she climbed into my lap, and we sat there for a while, and then we went into the bedroom together and woke up Jason. I nudged him gently, and when that didn't work, Daisy put her tongue up his nose, which worked every time.

"'Morning," I said as Jason squinted at me. "Get up, we're going to go and adopt a kitten."

"Wha!" said Jason, rubbing his eyes and shoving Daisy and her tongue away from his face.

"There was a kitten for adoption in the vet's office yesterday. Let's go adopt him." And Jason, who was always up for a new adventure with animals, which was one of the many things I loved about him, hopped out of bed and before we knew it we were on our way home with a brand-new little gray-and-white kitten we named Hamlet. Jason had wanted to call him Newman. And, as it turned out, that name would have been more appropriate.

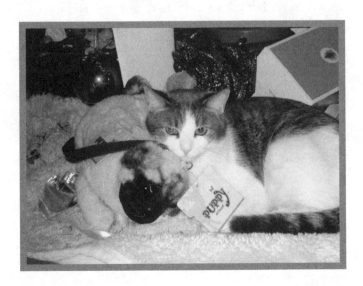

Hamlet, a Central Park rescue, was from the very first the most self-confident creature I have ever encountered. We sat him down in the middle of the living room to see what would happen. He immediately got up, walked right into the middle of the pug-puppy pile, and sat down and started to purr. It was as if he had been a part of the family all along and had just run out for a dish of milk or something. And Elvis, who has a huge heart but a brain the size of a grape, thought that he had a new baby, and began to lick Hamlet all over and fuss over him like a long-lost prodigal puppy.

Daisy, who had still been sitting shiva on the spot where Nick had left her, got up at last and climbed into the puppy bed with the new kitten, and life started up again.

"Well, we did it again," said Jason, as we sat on the couch watching the new kitten climb up the new drapes.

"Yeah," I said.

"Pretty great, isn't he?" Jason said and grinned at me.

"Yeah," I said, smiling despite myself.

"So, will you marry me?"

I just looked at him

"No really, will you marry me?" Jason said and then I swear he got on his knee, which made me feel awkward and wonderful all at the same time, and said again, "Beverly, will you marry me?"

And I said, "Yeah."

NICK PENNACCHINI

1988–2004

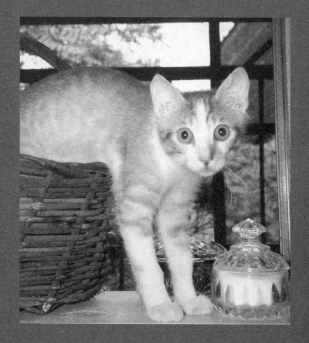

We love and miss you, Nicky!

Daisy says she's keeping your

favorite chair warm.

Ten

Fat
Daisy

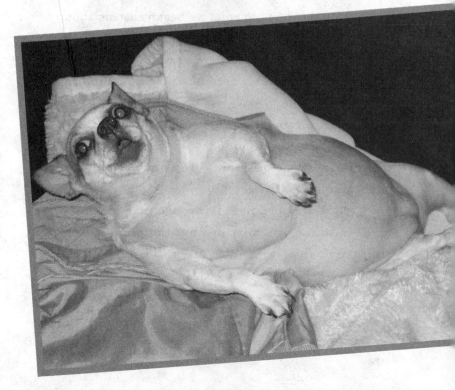

With Elvis's latest book, *Pugtherapy,* in the can and delivered to the publisher, and after convincing Elvis to go into semiretirement while he waited for the next big role, we began casting about for our next muse. She wasn't long in emerging. In fact, once we recognized her, we wondered how we could have missed her, because she was about as big as a double-wide.

The inspiration first came to us the day we noticed that Daisy was no longer just pleasingly plump. She wasn't cheerfully zaftig or adorably round or Rubenesque. Daisy was *fat.*

Well, I'd spoiled her all through the pregnancy, and while she was nursing. But the puppies were full-grown dogs now, and Daisy still hadn't lost the baby weight.

Plus, I think we were probably more aware of waistlines at that time. After all, we were now planning a wedding. Weddings involved wedding gowns, and Prada wedding suits, and worse yet, photographers. And all the dogs were in the wedding, including Daisy. And it was a *very* long aisle. So Daisy's girth was a good target for us to project our own bridal body image problems upon. And so of course, we fixated on her with intensity, and set to work.

At first we decided upon a sensible, relaxed, gradual approach to getting the weight off, which means we did little or nothing. This method, of course, failed entirely. In fact, far from dropping weight, she was now spilling over the sides of her princess bed and had outgrown even her fat sweaters. And one visit to the dressmaker to get fitted for my gown had assured me that Daisy wasn't the only one. So we resolved to go on a family diet, and lose the weight before the wedding. And we decided to do this project, just like we did everything else, together.

We embarked in our usual way. We went shopping. We bought Daisy a really cute new outfit. Then we bought ourselves one. And then we went food shopping. First we cut fats from our grocery list. Next it was carbs. We Sugar-Busted, South-Beached, and Slim-Fasted. And then we wrote a funny book about the whole process called *Fat Daisy*, during which we realized something that I think Daisy knew even way back in the puppy-adoption window.

Underneath all of that puppy fat, Daisy was a star. And she was even more of a natural than Elvis. Which really pissed Elvis off. The whole time Daisy was in front of the lens, Elvis pouted and howled, and eventually, we had to arrange to have somebody take him out so he wouldn't ruin Daisy's concentration.

Despite Elvis's ego, Daisy was hitting her stride, but the steps we were taking to get her and our weight off were coming up short. Basically, nothing was happening. After finally exhausting every reduced-calorie food on the market (of which there are startlingly few), without success, I began to get the idea that maybe something more than just what we were feeding Daisy and ourselves needed to change. But before I could figure out what that something was, life stepped in again to teach us the lesson the hard way, so we would never forget it.

One morning, I woke up and went into the kitchen to make breakfast, just like I do every morning. The puppies woke up and followed me, just like always. Only when I looked down for Daisy, she wasn't there. Daisy had followed me into the kitchen every morning since the very first day that we brought her home. So not seeing her wagging her tail at my feet the moment the can-opener began to buzz was very unsettling.

"Daisy!" I called, but no sleepy, fat Chihuahua emerged. I went back into the bedroom looking for her and found her, sitting on the edge of the bed, looking very upset.

"Come on, Daisy," I said, "puppy breakfast time." But Daisy didn't budge. What was going on? Daisy always woke up happy, because she knew breakfast was imminent. She always moved for food. But this morning she looked very subdued and glum, and she didn't move a muscle. She didn't even wag her tail or pick her head up. Something was obviously very wrong.

"Come on Daisy," I said, trying to disguise the rising panic in my voice. "Let's go have breakfast." Still nothing. So I picked her up and carried her into the living room. The other dogs rushed into the kitchen, tails wagging, begging for breakfast like they hadn't eaten in a week. I put Daisy on the floor so she could trot in after them, but the moment I put her down, Daisy's legs bucked. Somehow, between the night before and that morning, Daisy had lost the ability to walk.

"Jason, *JASON!*" I shouted, in yet another in the series of early morning, start-up-out-of-bed moments that characterized our life. Jason came stumbling sleepily from the bedroom to see what was wrong, and stubbed his toe on the sideboard. Thank God some things never changed.

"Daisy can't walk." He could see, even through the sleep in his eyes, that I was shaken up. He bent down and looked intently at Daisy.

"What's wrong, girl?" Jason bent down and gently set Daisy on her feet. Daisy tried to take a couple of steps just to please Jason, and then lay back down, looking miserable.

Jason looked at me with big saucer eyes. "What should we do?" he said then, his mouth dry and his voice catching. I understood. It's scary when an animal gets sick. It's so hard to know what to do for them, because they can't tell you what's wrong.

And of course, in situations like this, we had learned that there was really only one thing you could do. So I picked up the phone and dialed the dreaded vet tech. Only this time, when I explained what had happened to Daisy, they didn't sound quite so bored. Well, it wasn't a holiday. They told us to bring Daisy down right away. My heart started pounding. If we had gotten the vet techs rattled, something really awful must be happening to Daisy. So we bundled her up in her most slimming sweater and nestled her into her coziest sling, and rushed off to the vet's office to face the truth.

After an interminable cab ride, and the usual chorus of "*awww*"s, "*ooooh*"s, and the occasional snigger that Daisy always invites, our vet examined Daisy and then sat down, took off her gloves, and looked at us earnestly.

"Daisy is fat," she said.

"Yeah," Jason and I both mumbled, and looked at our feet.

"She never lost the puppy weight," Jason said, but the excuse just fell out onto the metal examining table and lay there. I think it even clanked when it hit the cold steel, and then rolled onto the floor.

"We've really been trying," I said helplessly. "We feed her reduced-calorie food, and I've been supplementing with vegetables. Well, except for a few treats." Our vet smiled and brought out a chart.

"This is the shape of a dog at the correct weight," she said. We looked down at the svelte, V-shaped doggie drawing at the top of the chart. Then she pointed to the drawing on the bottom of the bell curve. "And this," she said "is the shape of an obese dog." The obese doggie drawing looked a lot skinnier than Daisy. Jason and I looked at each other and gulped.

"And there's another problem," the vet said and turned Daisy on her back and extended one of her back legs. Daisy looked like her eyes were about to pop out of her head.

"Daisy has a luxated patella on both legs," she said, extending and contracting both knees. Daisy started to pant. "That means her knees are permanently out of joint. It's a congenital problem, but her weight is making things worse. You've got to get her weight down."

"Is she in pain?" I asked, looking at Daisy and wincing. I felt so guilty. This was my fault.

"I imagine that she's pretty uncomfortable," the vet said. "Just imagine walking with your knees out of joint."

"Is she going to walk again?" asked Jason, as usual charging in where I feared to tread.

"We can do surgery for the knees," she said, a little more gently now. I think she could see how bad we felt. "We have almost 100 percent success with the surgery, and Daisy will be as good as new and running around the way a dog her age should be. *But . . .*"

Uh oh, I thought to myself, here it comes.

"We can't do the surgery until she takes some of the weight off. She's too much of a risk for surgery, and also, at this weight, her knees would only go out again."

She paused for a moment while we took in the information. "Daisy is a very special dog," she said then. "She's got a lot to offer the world. Pet obesity is a big problem in this country. Who knows, maybe Daisy could become the very first canine fitness guru."

Then she gave Daisy a pat and went to get her a treat. "Here, Daisy, here's your last bite of fattening food for a very long time," she said. And Daisy, as if she understood and didn't want to miss her last empty calorie, wagged her tail weakly and gobbled the treat. I noticed that I felt instantly better the second Daisy ate something. I had somehow come to equate health with a healthy appetite.

"I'll give you a diet to start you out, and something to make Daisy more comfortable while she's losing the weight. But she needs to lose seven pounds."

"That's half her body weight," said Jason, horrified.

The vet smiled empathetically and stroked Daisy's

head. "Chihuahuas can live a very long time," she said, "but not like this."

And then I got serious.

We had to change, for Daisy. It was all up to us. After all, Daisy wasn't opening up the refrigerator and feeding herself. She wasn't climbing up on the counter and hitting "Frappe" on the shake-maker. If she was going to change, we were going to have to change as a family, and figure out how to express love without the use of empty calories.

Eleven

We Are Family

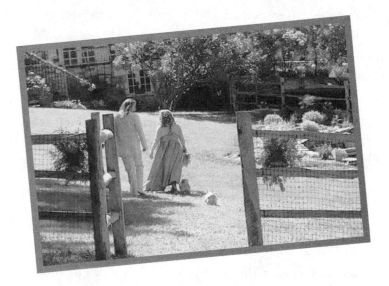

After just a month on the Happily Ever After Maintenance Plan, we were really beginning to see the difference in Daisy, and in ourselves. Although we had kind of secretly hoped that we would be sprinting through a field of clover in a bikini with wonderfully thin thighs in just thirty days, unfortunately, things just don't work that way in the real world. Pounds don't miraculously melt off people in a month, and they don't melt off teacup Chihuahuas, either. Let's just say, none of us was ready for our *Legally Blonde* audition . . . *yet*.

So okay, we weren't Reese Witherspoon. But some very important progress had been made. And if we'd learned one thing over the last few years, it was to focus on the positives. And one of our most important positives was the fact that Daisy was walking again. And in just one month, she had lost three whole pounds. And I had to have my wedding dress taken in, because I had lost eight inches.

Clearly, we were on to something. And we wanted to keep it up, but the wedding was barreling down upon us like a hydrangea-and-hyacinth-bedecked freight train, and we needed some flexibility with our plan, so we developed a short list that we could use as a guideline to get us through the hectic times and still have a happy ending.

Even afterward, when we had the leisure to settle down and get back to a more consistent routine and resume working toward our ideal, feeling-strong-and-good-about-life weight, these rules of thumb have served as a useful tool to help us remember what is at the heart of maintaining a beautiful and healthful life. So we wanted to share them with all of you, so that you, too, can rely on them when things get a little crazy.

As was par for the course with us by now, planning our wedding was a period crammed full of everything *but* wedding plans. Instead of picking our colors, and sampling wedding cakes, and registering for gifts, we were writing one book, doing publicity for a second book, keeping a vigilant eye on Daisy's legs and waistline, as well as our own, and believe it or not, fighting yet another court

Happily Ever After Maintenance Plan Short List

Develop and maintain a positive perspective.

Don't forget to breathe and laugh.

Avoid eating meals out of a can.

Eat meals together as a family as often as you can.

Eat plenty of fresh seasonal vegetables.

Taste your food, don't inhale it.

Don't eat stress. Choose organic meat, fish, eggs, and milk.

Make new friends and explore new places and new foods and new smells.

Consume artisanal products locally.

Eat a piece of fruit every once in a while and lay off the fries, already.

Watch your portions. Never eat anything that is bigger than your head.

Cooking should elevate and enhance your ingredients.

Try to make healthy choices at least 80 percent of the time.

Don't chase after parked cars.

battle to hold on to our rent-stabilized apartment. Sometimes living in New York City can be a very Sisyphean experience. You have to be willing to roll a lot of rocks uphill only to have them knocked back down to the bottom again by some sinister and ill-intentioned landlord looming far above and beyond you. It takes courage and a good law firm to pay under market in this town and get away with it. It's like living with a price on your head. But so far, the good guys had been winning, so we continued to trust in the justice and wisdom of the universe, as well as the New York City housing court.

We were also agonizing about how to break it to the owner of the historic inn we'd chosen to host our wedding weekend that our wedding party included four dogs. Our innkeeper didn't like dogs. In fact, her best friend had been killed by one when she was a child. I didn't have high hopes for our prospects. And it was very important for us to have the dogs with us. They were, after all, part of the family, and the wedding party. We'd even had flower garlands made for their harnesses. So we *had* to bring them. But it wasn't looking promising and I was having trouble working up the courage to ask.

And then somehow, miraculously, the way things suddenly coalesce out of the blue just when you really need them to, the innkeeper said yes, our friends and families arrived from hither and yon, and we packed up the gowns and the suits and the people and the puppies into the biggest SUV we could find, and led the longest rental car caravan we'd ever seen up to the Berkshire Mountains to make it legal.

And as many a bride and groom can attest to, when you are engaged in the process of making a fantasy come true, sometimes you hit a few snags along the way. First off, the dogs *hated* riding in cars. They were New York City dogs; it was a completely foreign experience to them, save for the occasional cab ride. And we had put them all in the same kennel in the far back of the behemoth of a buggy we'd rented to transport us to paradise, which did not make them happy at all. Elvis sounded like he was going to hyperventilate, Daisy was furious, Bert was a nervous wreck, and Buddha was perfectly fine, as usual. That puppy had really lived up to her name.

No doubt about it, traveling with puppies wasn't the bucolic drive through the country that we had anticipated. And even once we'd made it to the inn, and were safely behind closed doors, we spent most of our time trying to keep Elvis from permanently polluting the inn's pristine pinstripes and pine bedposts. We finally had to lock them all in the bathroom just to get a few minutes to relax.

But that night we had our rehearsal dinner with our families and friends, and didn't rehearse, and went to sleep with the puppies between us, or at least we did once the neighbors complained and the Stockbridge sheriff was called and the inn-keepers shut down the bar and threw Jason and his brothers out of the community gathering room. The Berkshires can, on occasion, be very Salem circa 1650. They are not keen on midnight revelry of any kind, even if it is taking place at nine thirty at night.

We woke up to a beautiful Berkshire morning. The sky was brilliant blue; the air held the promise of summer, but still had the crispness of a mountain spring. It was, in fact, 9/11 weather, although from that day forward when I look out in the morning on one of those brilliant blue days that herald the change of a season, I don't think of the Twin Towers falling, I think of our wedding day instead.

I woke up quite early to head off to the salon in Stockbridge with my best friend, Pam. Before I left, I put my wedding ring on the nightstand next to Jason and spent a moment looking at my young soon-to-be husband and the dogs all snoring soundly. At that moment, I felt like the luckiest woman in the world. Then I noticed that the pug had scratched Jason's cheek in his sleep. And it had left a nasty red mark, too. That wasn't going to make him happy.

"Don't forget to wake up for your hair appointment at eleven," I said, kissed his cheek, and then added, "and you better tell Kristopher to bring his concealer." Thank God, Jason's best man always traveled with a full MAC arsenal. Not to mention a pharmacy.

And then Pam knocked on the door and we headed off into the brand-new day.

Jason slept through his hair appointment.

And the wedding gown didn't fit.

And Elvis chewed through his flower garland. So did Bert.

And Daisy threw up on the worsted wool rug.

And Jason cried all the way down the aisle.

But thank God, Kristopher had remembered his concealer.

And when we finally arrived at the stand of old white birch trees at the edge of the stream that Jason to this day insists on calling a creek, which really pisses off the neighbors in Alford, despite all of the chills and spills and near-death experiences we had been through over the last few years, I knew we had all arrived safely right where we were supposed to be. And as the wind sang in the towering sugar maples that looked to me like God's broccoli florets, we promised to love and care for each other for the rest of our lives.

And as we made our way back up the aisle with the puppies running after us, including Daisy, and Frank Sinatra crooning "New York, New York" in the background, I knew that this was exactly what we were going to do, for as long as heaven and our health would allow.

Twelve

Fat Daisy's
Inner-Beauty Plan for
Puppies and
People

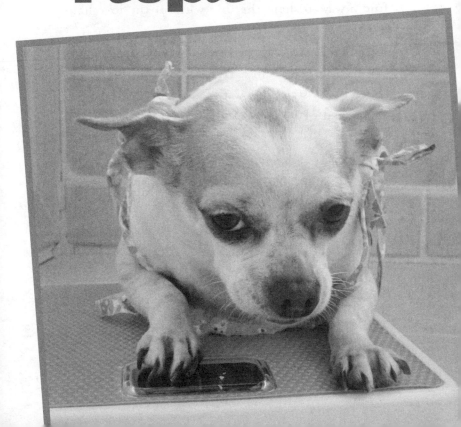

The very next day, we resolved as a family to improve our health, increase our happiness, and find a way to share the love without the love handles.

In the beginning, we focused primarily on Daisy, because she was in an extreme situation. So we followed a very strict diet with her which basically was comprised of 1/2 cup of vegetables and 1/4 cup of boiled chicken morning and night. And nothing else. Ever. For treats, we fed her raw carrots or apples. We kept her on this strict diet until she had lost a couple of pounds and was out of imminent danger.

Then, starting with the guidelines our vet had given us, we began to develop a more long-term, permanent lifestyle approach, and developed a plan that we could do together as a family to make sure that all of us would be able to dance the night away, not only at the wedding, but for happily ever after. And through much trial and error, some strategic interventions, advice, and encouragement from our kind vet, and more than a few late-night french-fry-and-Yummy-Chummies cravings, we came up with what we now call "The Happily Ever After Maintenance Plan," which has helped our whole family to look and feel our best, from the inside out, and for the rest of our lives.

It's important to note that this is *not* a diet plan. This is an Inner Beauty plan. Health and beauty are about more than calories and fat grams, pounds, and inches. So in addition to a menu for each day, we've also developed inner-strength-building exercises, inspirational thoughts designed to shift your perspective, and suggestions for ways that you and your dog can share your life and share your love, without loading up on empty calories. We've only covered two meals a day, because that's all your pet needs, so you'll be on your own for lunch. But we think, based on the other two meals that day, that you will be able to figure out the kinds of foods you'll want to be eating. And a good general rule of thumb is to go for the fruit and lay off the fries. It's really just common sense.

The philosophy of food embodied in this plan

is about feeding yourself and your pet fresh, organic, quality meals, in moderate portions and prepared in ways that elevate and enhance the nutritional value and flavor of nature's finest ingredients.

There is no dog food in this diet. Dog food as a general rule is very high in calories, and a lot of other things besides. Some labels read like a piece of PETA-sponsored performance art. And Daisy, who I swear could pick up weight just by standing next to a Happy Meal, really can't handle the carb-loaded by-products. This will obviously be more work for you. We think it's worth it. In our adventure with love, food, and dogs, we have found that enjoying healthful, beautiful, and delicious meals together, prepared with the best that you, the earth, and the seasons have to offer, is one of the very finest ways to share the love with your pets, your family, and yourself.

The menus in this plan are what worked for our family, and our Fat Daisy. They are meant as guidelines and suggestions to help you discover the kinds of healthful, quality food that your family enjoys, and that suit you and your dog's lifestyle, specific health needs, and metabolism. Some dogs have difficulty with a variety of foods; some dogs crave it. Some like peas, others like carrots; some want to eat only meat and potatoes every day, just like people. So this plan is intended to help you learn about your own and your pet's culinary preferences, and give you the guidelines and suggestions to work with your own appetites to develop a long-term and healthful plan of your own.

There are some ingredients that people can eat but your pets just can't tolerate. Dogs can't eat onions or pepper, or chocolate or grapes, for example. So we've avoided these ingredients for the most part in these recipes, and where they *are* included they are used for people portions only! Dogs aren't as dependent upon spice as we are.

In addition, we suggest that you check with your vet and your doctor before starting this or any fitness plan. The portions in this diet are designed for one person and one Fat Daisy. Portions are important, so be moderate. You and your dog should be eating until you are satisfied, not until you are full. There's a difference. We also recommend including a vitamin supplement, as well as Omega-3 and -6 fatty acids, with this plan.

Day 1

Inner-Beauty Thought for the Day:

I think dogs are the most amazing creatures; they give unconditional love. For me they are the role model for being alive.

—GILDA RADNER

Breakfast: Scrambled Eggs and Sunshine

The best way to dive in to any new project is to shine a little light on the situation. This breakfast will bring all the sunshine in and show you that you don't need hash browns to be happy.

HERE'S WHAT YOU'LL NEED:
1/2 cup poached wild organic salmon,
    flaked
1 tablespoon fresh dill
3 eggs
1 cup lowfat cottage cheese
1 tablespoon fresh parsley, minced
3/4 of a fresh cantaloupe

HERE'S HOW YOU DO IT: Poach salmon fillet in a covered sauté pan with the dill. Remove from the heat, cool, and pull apart into large flakes. Next, scramble all three eggs until firm but moist. Take the pan off the heat and mix in the cottage cheese and poached salmon. Sprinkle with fresh parsley and dill.

HOW TO SERVE YOURSELF: Arrange your sunshine eggs on your best china plate, because it is the first day of the rest of your life, after all, so break down and use the good dishes. Slice the melon into thin slices, or dice into bite-sized pieces and arrange alongside your eggs. Salt and pepper to taste.

HOW TO SERVE YOUR PUPPY: Dice the cantaloupe and mix in with the eggs, cottage cheese, and salmon. Serve at room temperature in your Daisy's best puppy bowl.

Inner-Beauty Regimen

Identify a theme song for you and your dog. It could be the same song, or different songs for each of you, but it should have special meaning and inspire you, and make you both feel beautiful when you listen to it while on an inspirational walk.

Dinner: Voluntary Simplicity Chicken

When you're trying to make a major lifestyle change, sometimes it's helpful to make a start by breaking things down and getting back to the basics. This recipe is a good reminder that less is more.

HERE'S WHAT YOU'LL NEED:
2 organic, cage-free chicken breasts on the
    bone
2 baked potatoes
1 tablespoon olive oil
Salt to taste
Pepper to taste (people portions only)
1 tablespoon fresh thyme
2 cups organic haricot vert

HERE'S HOW YOU DO IT: Place chicken breasts and potatoes on sheet pan, coat with olive oil, and sprinkle with salt, pepper (for humans only!), and fresh thyme. Bake at 375 degrees F for 30 to 40 minutes or until the chicken and the potato are done. Let the chicken rest for 10 minutes under some tinfoil. Trim and steam the haricot vert and salt lightly, or dry sauté with a little soy sauce.

HOW TO SERVE YOURSELF: Serve 1 chicken breast, 1/2 a baked potato, and plenty of haricot vert on a minimalist-inspired plate without a garnish. Reserve the remaining half chicken breast and half baked potato and 1 cup haricot vert for tomorrow's breakfast.

HOW TO SERVE YOUR DOG: Dice chicken, haricot vert, and a little of the potato, toss together, and serve at room temperature.

Fat Daisy's Inner-Strength Training

Take your dog for a walk, and when the road diverges in the wood, take the one less traveled by. You'll not only get some good exercise, but discover how many wonderful new things have been right around the corner all along. In the beginning, we carried Daisy around in her sling because she couldn't walk yet, but just the new surroundings seemed to excite her, and excitement burns calories. And so does carrying fifteen pounds of Fat Daisy on your shoulder!

Day 2

Inner-Beauty Thought for the Day:

Dogs laugh, but they laugh with their tails.

—MAX EASTMAN

Breakfast: Nonfat and Sassy Frittata

Just because you're on a weight loss plan doesn't mean you're not allowed to have fun.

HERE'S WHAT YOU'LL NEED:
Pam
4 strips turkey bacon, diced
Baked potato from last night's dinner,
    diced
1/2 cup broccoli, diced
Olive oil (optional)
3 eggs (or if you want to do egg whites only,
    5 egg whites)
1/3 cup nonfat milk
1/4 cup grated cheddar cheese
Salt to taste
Pepper (people portions only)

HERE'S HOW YOU DO IT: Spray a sauté pan with Pam, toss in diced turkey bacon and baked potato, and cook until the bacon and potatoes are brown and a little crispy. Add broccoli last and sauté until tender. Add a little olive oil if the mixture is dry. In a separate bowl, beat eggs and milk together and pour over the bacon and broccoli mixture. Top with grated cheddar, cover, and simmer on low. When frittata is firm, flip and brown on the other side for 2 to 3 minutes. Turn off heat, and cover.

HOW TO SERVE YOURSELF: Sprinkle with a dash of hot sauce, or some fresh ground salt and black pepper. Serve warm on a plate, garnished with some parsley or a little fresh fruit.

HOW TO SERVE YOUR DOG: Serve at room temperature, without the spice, in a bowl. If you are feeding a Fat Daisy of your own, only serve a very minute amount of bacon.

Inner-Beauty Regimen

When you're relaxing in front of the tube tonight with your favorite couchmate, instead of reaching for that Pup-peroni pizza, treat yourself and your puppy to a pedi and a pawdi. And don't be afraid of color!

Dinner: More for Us Muttballs

You can have three—they're small!

HERE'S WHAT YOU'LL NEED:
1/2 pound organic ground turkey
1/2 cup fresh whole wheat bread crumbs
1 organic cage-free egg
2 tablespoons olive oil
2 tablespoons parsley
Dash Worcestershire sauce
Salt to taste
Pam
1/2 cup flour, for dredging
1 cup organic chicken stock

HERE'S HOW YOU DO IT: Combine all the ingredients except the flour and the chicken stock in a large bowl, and blend with a fork. Don't overblend your meat; it makes for heavy meatballs! Form into small meatballs, roll in flour, and brown in a Dutch oven. When meatballs are brown on all sides, add the chicken stock, cover, and simmer on low until the meatballs are done (about 30 minutes).

HOW TO SERVE YOURSELF: Serve hot with a drizzle of the gravy on top, and a tossed salad on the side.

HOW TO SERVE YOUR DOG: Cool the muttballs and break them up in a little bowl so that your puppy doesn't wolf them down in one big schkorff. If your dog is allergic to wheat, which many dogs are, omit the bread crumbs.

Fat Daisy's Inner-Strength Training

After dinner, burn off a few of those calories by dancing with your dog. Work out a routine to your new theme song. In case you didn't know it, dogs have some really good moves. Try laughing with your tail in time to the music. It's great for the glutes, the abs, and the attitude.

Day 3

Inner-Beauty Thought for the Day:

The great pleasure of a dog is that you may make a fool of yourself with him and not only will he not scold you, but he will make a fool of himself too.

—SAMUEL BUTLER

Breakfast: Power Porridge

In a house full of dogs, some occasional fiber is a good thing. It's not too bad for you, either. Try it, you'll like it!

HERE'S WHAT YOU'LL NEED:
1 cup oatmeal
1/2 cup plain yogurt
1 ripe banana, sliced
6 ripe strawberries, sliced
3 tablespoons honey

HERE'S HOW YOU DO IT: Prepare oatmeal according to package instructions. You can even use instant oatmeal if you like, although Daisy prefers Irish steel-cut. She's become a real porridge snob.

HOW TO SERVE YOURSELF: Top oatmeal with yogurt and fresh fruit. Drizzle with honey and serve hot.

HOW TO SERVE YOUR DOG: Stir in yogurt and fresh fruit, and drizzle with a little honey. Serve at room temperature.

Inner-Beauty Regimen

Teach your dog a new trick. Then teach yourself one.

Dinner: The Whole Enchilada

Because this is your life, and this is your dinner, and you *can* eat it all.

HERE'S WHAT YOU'LL NEED:
1/2 pound organic ground chicken
1/2 cup brown rice

A little olive oil
1 cup organic chicken stock
A few saffron threads
1 cup fresh asparagus, diced
6 small corn tortillas
1/4 cup grated Reggiano
Salt to taste

HERE'S HOW YOU DO IT: Brown the chicken and the rice in a little olive oil in a Dutch oven until lightly browned. Add the chicken stock and saffron threads, cover, and simmer on low for 15 minutes. Add the asparagus, fluff into the rice, then recover and simmer for another 15 minutes or until the chicken is done and the rice is tender. Spoon the rice and meat into corn tortillas, roll, cover in broth, and top with grated Reggiano. Salt to taste.

HOW TO SERVE YOURSELF: Serve hot on a fiesta-inspired charger.

HOW TO SERVE YOUR DOG: Allow the enchiladas to cool and cut into slices. Slices are great the next day for a festive and low-calorie reward for doing something cute. If your dog is allergic to wheat, or seriously overweight, omit the corn tortillas.

Fat Daisy's Inner-Strength Training

Instead of hopping in the car, do what errands you can on foot and take your dog along with you. It's good for the planet, saves on gas, encourages you to shop locally, you'll both get more exercise, and you'll be amazed at how many neighbors you meet along the way.

Day 4

Fat Daisy's Inner-Beauty Thought for the Day:

*Until one has loved an animal, a part of one's soul remains
unawakened.*

—ANATOLE FRANCE

Breakfast: The Big Apple

It's a brand-new day. Wake up and smell the apple
sausage.

HERE'S WHAT YOU'LL NEED:
3 chicken and apple sausages
A little olive oil
2 apples cored, peeled, and
      sliced
Sprinkle of salt, brown sugar, fresh nutmeg,
      and cinnamon
1/4 cup apple cider

HERE'S HOW YOU DO IT: Brown your sausages in a sauté pan in a little
olive oil. Toss the apples with each sprinkle of salt, brown sugar, fresh
nutmeg, and cinnamon. When sausages are browned on all sides, pour
in the cider, cover, and simmer for 15 minutes.

HOW TO SERVE YOURSELF: Spoon the apple slices to make a bed on a
good-quality, prairie-inspired plate and arrange sausages on top of the
apples.

HOW TO SERVE YOUR DOG: Wait until the mixture is cool, then slice sausages into pieces and mix with the apple slices in a bowl. If your dog is seriously overweight, omit the brown sugar.

Inner-Beauty Regimen

Today, experiment with ways to say "I love you" to your dog, and yourself, without using food treats.

Dinner: The Cuddle Kebab

HERE'S WHAT YOU'LL NEED:
jasmine rice
1 pound lamb, cubed
2 medium-sized zucchinis
1 medium-sized eggplant, cubed
Cherry tomatoes, onions, peppers
    (for people kebabs only)
Wood kebab skewers, soaked in water
Basil leaves
Mint leaves
Olive oil
Salt, (and pepper for the people kebabs)

HERE'S HOW YOU DO IT: Cook your jasmine rice according to the directions on the package and set aside. Cut up your lamb and veggies and arrange on skewers. For the dogs, alternate lamb, zucchini, and eggplant along with the basil and mint leaves. On the people kebabs, you can also add in cherry tomatoes, onions, and green peppers. Brush with olive oil, salt, and grill until tender.

HOW TO SERVE YOURSELF: Take the vegetables and meat off your kebab and arrange on a bed of jasmine rice on a festive plate.

HOW TO SERVE YOUR DOG: Allow to cool, then toss the puppy kebabs with the jasmine rice in your dog's most colorful bowl. If your dog needs to drop a few kebabs, eliminate the rice.

Fat Daisy's Inner-Strength Training

Spend a half hour playing a contact sport with your dog. Toss a ball, throw a Frisbee, or chuck a stick, then chase your dog down and try to get it back! Not only will the aerobic activity burn off calories for you both, but it will also strengthen the relationship between you and your best friend.

Day 5

Inner-Beauty Thought for the Day:

Dogs are not our whole life, but they make our lives whole.

—ROGER CARAS

Breakfast: Everything's Coming up Carrots

This light and airy start to the day is good for you and your dog's waistline, as well as your vision.

Preheat the oven to 350 degrees F.

HERE'S WHAT YOU'LL NEED:
1 1/2 pounds carrots, sliced
3 large eggs
1/2 cup dark brown sugar
4 tablespoons butter, at room temperature
1/4 cup all-purpose flour
1/4 cup milk
2 tablespoons orange juice
Zest of 1/2 orange
3/4 teaspoon baking powder
Dash salt, cinnamon, and nutmeg

HERE'S HOW YOU DO IT: Bring a large pot of water to a boil, add the carrots, and cook until tender, about 15 minutes; drain. Combine the carrots with the remaining ingredients in a food processor and hit puree until smooth. Spoon into a greased soufflé dish or casserole dish and bake for about an hour, until lightly browned.

HOW TO SERVE YOURSELF: Spoon onto a plate and top with a few pecans and a little maple syrup and fresh ground black pepper.

HOW TO SERVE YOUR DOG: Allow to cool and serve plain.

Fat Daisy's Inner-Beauty Regimen

Massage a little carrot oil into your scalp and your dog's coat. You'll be amazed at how silky your hair becomes, and spending a few extra moments taking care of you and your puppy sets you up to have a good day where you remember to take the extra time it takes to meet your own needs, in addition to everyone else's.

Dinner: Taking-Care-of-Ourselves
Tuna and Snow Peas

This dish is quick, easy, and delicious, leaving you more time to cuddle with your puppy.

HERE'S WHAT YOU'LL NEED:
1/2 pound organic tuna loin (whole)
Sesame seeds
Olive oil or sesame oil
1/2 pound snow peas
Soy sauce
Wasabi (people portions only)

HERE'S HOW YOU DO IT: Roll the tuna loin in sesame seeds and grill at a very high temperature in a little olive or sesame oil, whichever you prefer, until it is seared on all sides and red in the middle. Set aside. Trim your snow peas and place in a very hot pan for just a moment, tossing frequently. Add a dash of soy sauce, dry sauté for another minute, then remove from heat when the beans begin to shrivel slightly.

HOW TO SERVE YOURSELF: Slice the loin into thin slices and lay on a square, Asian-inspired white plate. Arrange the beans next to the tuna and serve with a sauce made from soy sauce and wasabi. This dish is best eaten with chopsticks.

HOW TO SERVE YOUR DOG: Allow to cool. Cut up tuna and beans and serve in a square, Asian-inspired white dog bowl. Do not expect your dog to use chopsticks.

Fat Daisy's Inner-Strength Training

Run up and down a flight of stairs ten times with your dog and see who gets nowhere quickest! This exercise is not only good aerobic activity, but reminds you that no matter where you go, there you are. So take your time and enjoy the climb.

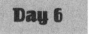

Inner-Beauty Thought for the Day:

If you think dogs can't count, try putting three dog biscuits in your pocket and then giving Fido only two of them.

—PHIL PASTORET

Breakfast: Pups in the Hole

This is like a little bit of puppy love served on toast.

HERE'S WHAT YOU'LL NEED:
4 slices whole wheat bread
1 tablespoon butter
4 eggs

HERE'S HOW YOU DO IT: Toast the slices of whole wheat bread and remove crusts, then, with a biscuit cutter, cut out a hole in the middle of each, and butter the toast lightly. Next, poach the eggs and drop one egg in each hole.

HOW TO SERVE YOURSELF: Serve hot. Salt and pepper to taste.

HOW TO SERVE YOUR DOG: Serve cool, and then cut up the eggs and toast so your dog doesn't eat breakfast in two quick bites. If your dog is allergic to wheat, substitute a ground turkey patty with a hole in the middle. Brown and fill with the poached egg.

Fat Daisy's Inner-Beauty Regimen

Read a book to your dog. He may not be able to understand the plot line, but he can read the love that's between the lines, and the more you talk to your dog, the more he understands. Plus, it's a way to make sure that you spend a few minutes reading a book, just for the pleasure of it.

Dinner: Say It with Stir-Fry

This delicious and nutritious meal will become a favorite way to say "I love you" with healthy food.

HERE'S WHAT YOU'LL NEED:
2 tablespoons olive oil
1/2 pound beef sirloin or eye round,
      sliced 1/4-inch thick
2 cups fresh snow peas
1 cup broccoli florets
2 cups asparagus spears, cut in quarters
2 cups sliced bok choi
1/4 cup water
2 tablespoons low-sodium soy sauce
1/4 cup orange juice
2 tablespoons raspberry vinegar
1 1/2 teaspoons cornstarch, dissolved in
      1/4 cup water

HERE'S HOW YOU DO IT: In a large sauté pan, or a wok, heat half of the oil on high heat, add the beef, and cook until just brown. Remove to a plate, cover, and set aside. Reduce heat to medium, add the remaining half of the oil, and add the vegetables. Cook for 3 to 4 minutes or until vegetables are beginning to soften. Then, add the remainder of the ingredients and the beef and stir until sauce is slightly thickened and beef is heated through.

HOW TO SERVE YOURSELF: Drizzle with a little sesame oil, and sprinkle with a little ground red pepper. Serve in a rice bowl, with chopsticks.

HOW TO SERVE YOUR DOG: Allow to cool and serve in a rice bowl, without chopsticks.

Fat Daisy's Inner-Strength Training

Take your dog on a scavenger hunt and collect something that you can put to use later. If it's autumn, go to the park and collect acorns, then use them as a decorative filling in a glass vase to hold flowers in place. Or collect red maple leaves and come home and press them. If it's winter, go in search of dried seed pods to make a decorative arrangement for your dinner table. You'll be amazed at the natural treasures you can find together, even in the middle of a big city.

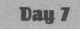

Inner-Beauty Thought for the Day:

Happiness is a warm puppy.

—CHARLES M. SCHULZ

Breakfast: Snausage Scramble

This is a hearty scramble that will stick to your ribs and keep you and your pup firing on all cylinders all day long, no matter how cold the weather. You can substitute pork sausage, if you prefer. I've suggested turkey, as it's leaner and meaner.

HERE'S WHAT YOU'LL NEED:
6 turkey breakfast sausages
3 eggs (or egg whites, if you prefer)
1/4 teaspoon dried thyme
Salt
1/4 cup nonfat milk
Pam

HERE'S HOW YOU DO IT: Bake your sausage until done. Next, whisk your eggs, thyme, salt, and nonfat milk in a bowl. Spray a sauté pan with Pam, and add the egg mixture. Then cut the sausage up into bite-sized pieces and scramble along with the eggs.

HOW TO SERVE YOURSELF: Serve hot on a plate with a little cracked pepper. You can also serve a tossed salad on the side, if you are extra hungry.

HOW TO SERVE YOUR DOG: Serve cool in a bowl. You can add a little cottage cheese, too, if your dog is extra hungry.

Fat Daisy's Inner-Beauty Regimen

Brush your hair for one hundred strokes until it shines. Then do the same thing for your puppy.

Dinner: Turkeylicious

Baking a turkey breast is a great way to keep you and your dog fed easily and quickly for multiple meals. Turkey is a superfood for both man and beast, so it's great to have around for treats, too, and snacks when you just can't resist. The calming properties of tryptophan don't hurt, either!

Preheat oven to 375 degrees F.

HERE'S WHAT YOU'LL NEED:
1 whole turkey breast
4 tablespoons olive oil
2 teaspoons salt
2 tablespoons fresh thyme
1 lemon (including zest)
1 apple
2 medium zucchinis, thinly sliced
8 organic heirloom cherry tomatoes

HERE'S HOW YOU DO IT: Wash and dry your turkey. Place in a roasting pan, and slather with the olive oil and salt, fresh thyme, and the zest of 1 lemon. Slice lemon and apple in half and place in the cavity of the breast, and roast until fully cooked. When the turkey is done, take out of the oven, cover with foil, and let it rest for about 15 minutes before carving. While your turkey rests, toss the zucchini slices and cherry tomatoes in olive oil, and roast until the tomatoes pop.

HOW TO SERVE YOURSELF: Carve the turkey and serve hot with the tomatoes and zucchini on a plate that is normally reserved for holidays.

HOW TO SERVE YOUR DOG: Carve smaller pieces of turkey and mix with the zucchini, and serve on a beautiful plate.

Fat Daisy's Inner-Strength Training

Plant a window garden with herbs and greens that are good for you and your puppy. Grow some parsley, oregano, thyme, and sage. They all grow very well in a sunny window box. And plant some wheat grass for your puppy—it's a great digestive aid. Gardening is terrific exercise, fresh herbs add a whole lot of flavor with very few calories, and a blade of grass a day keeps the vet away!

Day 8

Inner-Beauty Thought for the Day:

A dog is one of the remaining reasons why some people can be persuaded to go for a walk.

—O. A. BATTISTA

Breakfast: The Bottomless Quiche

This all-filling quiche will fill you both up without filling you out.

Preheat oven to 350 degrees F.

HERE'S WHAT YOU'LL NEED:
6 eggs
1/4 cup nonfat milk

Salt
Fresh parsley
1/2 cup Cheddar cheese
1/2 cup diced ham
1 cup steamed broccoli

HERE'S HOW YOU DO IT: Whisk eggs, milk, salt, and parsley in a bowl, and pour into a greased baking pan or pie plate. Add cheese, ham, and broccoli, and bake until puffy and golden brown.

HOW TO SERVE YOURSELF: Serve hot with green leaf salad and vinaigrette on the side.

HOW TO SERVE YOUR DOG: Serve at room temperature in a sunny-looking bowl. You can garnish with a little fresh fruit, like a few apple slices, if your puppy wants a little more color.

Fat Daisy's Inner-Beauty Regimen

Look at your dog for five minutes and try to memorize everything that you see. What color are your dog's eyes? What color eyelashes and whiskers does your dog have? Notice as many details as you can, then close your eyes and see how much you remember. Then open your eyes back up and see how accurate you were. Not only is this a great way to spend some quality time with your dog, and to notice any bumps or lumps that might need attention, but it reminds you to pay attention to the small details in life, because they make all the difference.

Dinner: Turkey Clubs

Everybody knows the best thing about a turkey dinner is the sandwiches you make with the leftovers.

HERE'S WHAT YOU'LL NEED:
Whole grain bread
1 tablespoon butter or lowfat mayonnaise
Slices of turkey bacon or uncured regular
     bacon with no nitrites
Slices of leftover turkey
Lettuce and tomato
Dash of salt

HERE'S HOW YOU DO IT: Coat good whole-grain bread with butter or lowfat mayonnaise, cook up a few slices of turkey bacon, and slap it on that bread, with slices of turkey and lettuce and tomatoes, and a dash of salt.

HOW TO SERVE YOURSELF: Slice diagonally, add pepper, if you like, and serve on a rectangular plate with a pickle or a green leaf salad.

HOW TO SERVE YOUR DOG:. Deconstruct the sandwich and serve in a bowl. If your dog has wheat allergies, or is looking a little paunchy around the Pope's nose, omit the bread and mayo.

Fat Daisy's Inner-Strength Training

Chase your puppy around the yard or the living room for ten or fifteen minutes. It's a good aerobic activity for you both!

Inner-Beauty Thought for the Day:

To sit with a dog on a hillside on a glorious afternoon is to be back in Eden, where doing nothing was not boring—it was peace.

—MILAN KUNDERA

Breakfast: Self-Esteem Salmon, Three Ways

Serve this breakfast and imagine yourself Sunday-brunching at Cipriani with a peach Bellini and a Chihuahua in your purse, and see if you both don't feel a lot better about yourselves afterward.

HERE'S WHAT YOU'LL NEED:
1 pound wild salmon and 1/2 pound
    smoked salmon
Juice and zest of 1 lemon and 1 lime
1/2 cup reduced-fat sour cream
1/2 cup fresh dill
1/2 teaspoon salt
1/4 teaspoon fresh ground black pepper
    (people portions only)
1/4 cup mustard
3 tablespoons honey
2 tablespoons champagne vinegar
4 tablespoons olive oil
1/2 cup diced celery

HERE'S HOW YOU DO IT:
First Way: Poach 1/2 pound of wild salmon in water with the juice of half a lemon and a dash of salt, and chill. For the sauce, mix 1/2 cup reduced-fat

sour cream with 1/4 cup minced fresh dill, 1/4 teaspoon of lemon zest, a dash of salt, and for people, a pinch of black pepper.

Second Way: Arrange smoked salmon in florets on a wooden plank. For the sauce, mix mustard, honey, vinegar, remaining fresh dill, and 1 tablespoon olive oil in a bowl, and whisk until well mixed and shiny.

Third Way: Cut 1/2 pound of the wild salmon into 1/4-inch cubes and place in a bowl. Add 3 tablespoons olive oil, zest and juice of 1 lime, 1/4 teaspoon salt, and for people, 1 teaspoon red pepper sauce, along with the diced celery, and marinate for half an hour to let flavors blend.

HOW TO SERVE YOURSELF: Serve your salmon three ways on a colorful rectangle, a wooden plank, or beautiful hardwood carving board. Serve the poached salmon with the sour cream and dill sauce in one corner, the smoked salmon and honey mustard sauce in another, and finally the salmon tartar in the center, with a few pepperoncino flakes sprinkled on top. Side dress with pumpernickel bread and quick-cooked asparagus that is still crispy.

HOW TO SERVE YOUR DOG: Serve your dog all three kinds of salmon, separated on a plate, and let him taste them each separately. Dogs eat more slowly when they have to move from one pile to the next. Serve with diced asparagus arranged in between the three dishes like a puppy palate cleanser. Go easy on the mustard sauce for your pooch, though— maybe just a little taste to wake up his palate.

Fat Daisy's Inner-Beauty Regimen

Sit with your dog for fifteen minutes and try to see the world through your pet's eyes. Be very quiet, don't move much, and try to notice what your dog notices: the sound of a leaf falling, a bird singing outside your window, your own breathing, or the beating of your heart. You will be amazed what you can learn about relaxation from your best friend, just by sitting quietly side by side and doing nothing at all.

Dinner: Love Yourself Pork Loin with Love Apples and Roasted Fingerlings

Preheat oven to 400 degrees F.

HERE'S WHAT YOU'LL NEED:
4 teaspoons Dijon mustard
2 tablespoons good olive oil
1 teaspoon ground fennel seed
1 pork tenderloin
2 apples, cut in half and cored
4 organic fingerling potatoes
3 more tablespoons good olive oil
Kosher salt
3 cups chicken stock

HERE'S HOW YOU DO IT: Make a paste with the mustard, olive oil, and fennel seed. Rub the paste over your tenderloin and place in a pan. Place the apples and fingerlings next to the tenderloin, drizzle with olive oil and salt, and roast until the internal temperature of the pork reaches 140 degrees F and the potatoes and apples are tender. Pour off jus and cover. Mix the jus with chicken stock and reduce by half.

HOW TO SERVE YOURSELF: Slice the tenderloin in half-inch slices and lay on a plate with the fingerlings and apple halves. Drizzle with jus, add ground pepper if you like, and serve piping hot.

HOW TO SERVE YOUR DOG: Slice the tenderloin in half-inch slices, then cut into chunks, along with the potatoes and apples, and serve in a bowl at room temperature.

Fat Daisy's Inner-Strength Training

Today, when you walk your dog, go a little farther and a little faster than you did yesterday. Then tomorrow, go a little farther and a little faster than that.

Day 10

Inner Beauty Thought for the Day:

I care not for a man's religion whose dog and cat are not the better for it.

—ABRAHAM LINCOLN

Breakfast: I Am Not a Crab Cakes

It's impossible for people or puppies to be in a bad mood when you start your day with a breakfast like this.

HERE'S WHAT YOU'LL NEED:
2 tablespoons unsalted butter
2 tablespoons olive oil
1 1/2 cups celery (4 stalks), small-diced
1/2 cup red bell pepper (1 small pepper),
     small-diced
1/2 cup yellow bell pepper (1 small pepper),
     small-diced
1/4 cup fresh flat-leaf parsley, minced

1 tablespoon capers, drained
1/2 teaspoon Worcestershire Sauce
1 1/2 teaspoons Old Bay
Zest of 1 lemon
1/2 teaspoon kosher salt
1/2 pound lump crabmeat, drained and
    picked to remove shells
1/2 cup plain dry bread crumbs
1/2 cup good lowfat mayonnaise
2 teaspoons Dijon mustard
2 extra-large eggs, lightly beaten
4 more tablespoons unsalted butter
1/4 cup more olive oil

HERE'S HOW YOU DO IT: Place the 2 tablespoons butter, 2 tablespoons oil, celery, red and yellow bell peppers, parsley, capers, Worcestershire sauce, Old Bay, lemon zest, and salt in a large sauté pan over medium-low heat, and cook until the vegetables are soft. Cool to room temperature. In a large bowl, break the lump crabmeat into small pieces and toss with the bread crumbs, mayonnaise, mustard, and eggs. Add the cooked vegetables, blend, and let sit in the refrigerator for about half an hour until the mixture firms up. Then shape into patties and fry in the additional butter and oil until browned on each side.

HOW TO SERVE YOURSELF: Put two cakes on a plate with a little fresh salsa, and garnish with parsley, corn salad, or a green salad. Or you can put a poached egg on top. Serve hot with a little fresh ground black pepper on top and make it into a Crab Benedict.

HOW TO SERVE YOUR DOG: Allow crab cakes to cool, break up, and serve in a bowl at room temperature. Puppies like Crab Benedict, too.

Fat Daisy's Inner-Beauty Regimen

It's been a week, so it's time for a new pedi and pawdi, only this time, try to exercise a little more color courage.

Dinner: World Peace Parmesan Chicken

Because if everybody ate like this, there would be no more reason to fight.

HERE'S WHAT YOU'LL NEED:
2 boneless, skinless chicken breasts
1/4 cup all-purpose flour
Dash kosher salt
1 egg
1 tablespoon water
1/4 cup dry bread crumbs
1/4 cup freshly grated Parmesan
1 tablespoon unsalted butter
1 tablespoon good olive oil
Mixed greens such as mesclun, endive,
 arugula, radicchio, and Bibb lettuce. A
 few nasturtiums or pansies are also
 nice for color, and completely edible
 and delicious.
Lemon vinaigrette

HERE'S HOW YOU DO IT: Pound the chicken breasts until they are about 1/4-inch thick. In a separate bowl, combine the flour and salt. In another bowl, whisk the egg and water, and in a third bowl, combine the bread crumbs and Parmesan cheese. Dip your chicken first in the flour, then in the egg, and then in the bread crumbs and cheese, and set on a plate in the refrigerator to set up. Next, heat 1 tablespoon of butter and 1 tablespoon of olive oil in a large sauté pan and cook the cutlets on medium to low heat until cooked through. Toss the salad greens with lemon vinaigrette or a lowfat Italian dressing.

HOW TO SERVE YOURSELF: Place a hot cutlet on a bed of salad and sprinkle with a little extra cheese.

HOW TO SERVE YOUR DOG: Cut up a cutlet and toss with the greens. Serve at room temperature in a salad bowl.

HOW TO MAKE A LIGHT LEMON VINAIGRETTE: In a small bowl, whisk together 1/4 cup freshly squeezed lemon juice (2 lemons), 1/2 cup good olive oil, 1/2 teaspoon kosher salt, and 1/4 teaspoon freshly ground black pepper.

Fat Daisy's Inner Strength Training

Find something that you and your puppy can do for a puppy or person who is less fortunate than you are. Donate to the Humane Society, volunteer to take a dog at a shelter for a walk, look into training your puppy as a therapy dog, or just go for a walk together and bring a smile to somebody who needs it.

Day 11

Inner-Beauty Thought for the Day:

Dogs lead a nice life. You never see a dog with a wristwatch.

—GEORGE CARLIN

Breakfast: Personal Best Egg Salad and Salmon Tartines

These are perfect to serve at a pooch party for your friends and their bitches who brunch. Very ladylike, but still filling and delicious, and you can eat them with your fingers.

HERE'S WHAT YOU'LL NEED:
6 extra-large eggs
1/3 cup good lowfat mayonnaise
1/2 teaspoon mustard
1/2 tablespoon minced fresh dill
Dash celery seed
1/2 teaspoon kosher salt
1/2 cup celery, diced
1 slice whole-grain bread
Olive oil
4 slices good smoked salmon

HERE'S HOW YOU DO IT: Hard boil your eggs and cool to room temperature. Peel the eggs and place in a food processor and pulse until the eggs are in small pieces about the size of large peas. Don't overpulse the eggs or they will turn into mush. Place the chopped eggs into a bowl and add the mayo, mustard, dill, celery seed, salt, and celery, and toss lightly with a fork. Again, be careful—nobody likes a pureed salad. Next, slice four slices of bread and brush with olive oil, salt lightly, and broil until lightly toasted. Lay a slice of salmon on each piece of bread, cover with egg salad, and garnish with dill.

HOW TO SERVE YOURSELF: Serve on an elegant luncheon plate with fresh dill sprigs and some freshly cracked pepper.

HOW TO SERVE YOUR DOG: Cut up into bite-sized pieces and serve on a tasteful plate. If your dog is seriously overweight or allergic to wheat, serve without the bread.

Fat Daisy's Inner-Beauty Regimen

Cultivate some fashion courage. Go shopping for new outfits with your puppy, and buy something for you both that you normally would never wear. You'll be amazed what you discover when you break out of your look nook.

Dinner: Because You're Special Fillet with Once in a While Fries

Let your puppys know how special he is to you with this lavish spread, which even includes a few matchstick fries, because you can do whatever you want, as long as it's only once in a while.

HERE'S WHAT YOU'LL NEED:
Kosher salt
2 filet mignon, 3/4-inch thick
1 1/2 cups vegetable oil
1 russet potato
1/3 teaspoon anchovy paste
Fresh rosemary, minced
1/4 cup olive oil

HERE'S HOW TO DO IT: Salt the filet mignon and allow to sit at room temperature for half an hour. Heat the vegetable oil in a sauté pan to 340 degrees F. Cut your potato into matchsticks and submerge in cold water and salt. When your oil reaches temperature, place the matchsticks into the hot oil. When they are well browned, drain on a paper towel, then place them on a cookie sheet, salt, and put them in the oven on medium heat. Heat a grill pan until it's very hot. Place your filets on the skillet and sear for 2 minutes on each side. Reduce heat to medium and cook for another 4 to 6 minutes. Remove from the grill pan. Next, mix the anchovy paste and minced fresh rosemary with the olive oil. Make sure to bruise the rosemary in the oil, then pour over the meat, cover with foil, and allow to rest for 10 minutes before serving.

HOW TO SERVE YOURSELF: Serve your filet mignon on a plate with matchstick fries and a mixed green salad. Drizzle some rosemary and anchovy oil over the top, and add freshly ground pepper, if you like.

HOW TO SERVE YOUR DOG: Slice and dice some of the filet mignon, toss in a few fries and greens, and serve in your dog's best bowl, then put the rest of the steak in a doggy bag for steak and eggs tomorrow morning.

Fat Daisy's Inner-Strength Training

Teach your dog a dance. Then let your dog teach you one.

Day 12

Inner-Beauty Thought for the Day:

Why, that dog is practically a Phi Beta Kappa. She can sit up and beg, and she can give her paw—I don't say she will, but she can.

—DOROTHY PARKER

Breakfast: Better the Second Time Around
Steak and Eggs

Because this meat really does look good in the morning.

HERE'S WHAT YOU'LL NEED:
2 tablespoons butter
Last night's leftover filet mignon
3 eggs
Salt

HERE'S HOW YOU DO IT: Melt 1 tablespoon butter in a skillet, throw your steak in the pan, and bring to temperature, then transfer to a plate and cover with foil. Next, melt another tablespoon of butter, and cook your eggs sunny side up. Sprinkle with the salt before serving.

HOW TO SERVE YOURSELF: Slice the meat in thin slices and serve with eggs, fresh cracked pepper, if you like, and a little ketchup or Tabasco sauce.

HOW TO SERVE YOUR DOG: Do Fido a favor and leave out the Tabasco sauce!

Fat Daisy's Inner-Beauty Regimen

Brainstorm some new ways to reduce your carbon paw-print, and then put them into practice.

Dinner: Friends for Life Lemon Fusilli with Broccoli and Chicken

Trust us, this dish will inspire loyalty. Once you've eaten this, you'll want to eat it again and again and again.

HERE'S WHAT YOU'LL NEED:
1 tablespoon good olive oil
1/2 pound boneless white chicken, cut into
    small pieces
1 cup fat-free half-and-half

2 lemons, juice and zest
Kosher salt
1 bunch broccoli
1/2 pound whole wheat fusilli
1/2 pound baby arugula
1/4 cup freshly grated Parmesan
1/2 pint grape or cherry tomatoes, halved

HERE'S HOW YOU DO IT: Heat the olive oil in a medium saucepan over medium heat, add the chicken, and cook until tender. Add the half-and-half, the zest of 2 lemons, the juice of 2 lemons, and 2 teaspoons of salt. Bring to a boil, then lower the heat and simmer for 15 to 20 minutes, until the liquid starts to thicken.

Meanwhile, cut the broccoli in florets and steam in a pot of boiling salted water for 3 to 5 minutes, until tender but still firm. Drain the broccoli and plunge into a cold water bath, then set aside.

Next, cook your pasta according to the directions on the package and drain when it is al dente. Put the pasta back in the pot, add your half-and-half mixture, and cook over medium-low heat until the sauce has been absorbed. Pour the pasta into a large bowl, add the arugula, Parmesan, tomatoes, and cooked broccoli, and toss well with a little salt.

HOW TO SERVE YOURSELF: Mince and toast one clove of garlic and toss into your serving, then serve a small portion in a Tuscan bowl with some freshly cracked pepper.

HOW TO SERVE YOUR DOG: Serve at room temperature without the garlic and black pepper.

Fat Daisy's Inner-Strength Training

Learn a new language and then teach your dog to obey commands in your new tongue.

Inner-Beauty Thought for the Day:

Some of my best leading men have been dogs and horses.

—ELIZABETH TAYLOR

Breakfast: Good for You Both Granola Sundae

Preheat the oven to 350 degrees F.

HERE'S WHAT YOU'LL NEED:
1 cup steel-cut Irish oats
1/2 cup sweetened, shredded coconut
1/2 cup sliced or slivered almonds
3 tablespoons vegetable oil
2 tablespoons good honey
8 to 10 strawberries
1/2 cup blueberries
8 to 10 raspberries
2 cups plain yogurt

HERE'S HOW YOU DO IT: Toss the oats, coconut, almonds, oil, and honey together in a large bowl, pour onto a sheet pan, and bake, turning occasionally, until the mixture turns a nice, even golden brown, about 20 minutes. Remove the granola from the oven, stir it around so it doesn't stick to the pan, then allow to cool completely. Next, combine with the strawberries, blueberries, and raspberries in a bowl. Serve with the yogurt (see below).

HOW TO SERVE YOURSELF: In a sundae glass, layer first the fruit, then the yogurt, and finally the granola, alternating layers until the glass is way more than half full.

HOW TO SERVE YOUR DOG: Combine the yogurt, fruit, and granola in a sundae dish. You can layer it if you like, but chances are your dog is going to eat it all in one big slurp.

Fat Daisy's Inner-Beauty Regimen

Grab your pup and get up off of that thing, and dance 'til you feel better.

Dinner: Sunday Afternoon Roast

When you're eating this good, every day feels like Sunday. This recipe for rib roast works perfectly every time, which is nothing short of a miracle.

Preheat the oven to 500 degrees F.

HERE'S WHAT YOU'LL NEED:
1 (3-rib) standing rib roast
1 tablespoon kosher salt
1 large bunch asparagus
1 tablespoon olive oil
1 tablespoon balsamic vinegar
1/4 cup grated Grana Padano

HERE'S HOW YOU DO IT: Bring your roast to room temperature and rub with salt. Place the roast in a large roasting pan, bone side down, and roast for 45 minutes at 500 degrees F. Then, turn the oven down to 325 and roast for another 30 minutes; then, finally, increase the temperature to 450, and roast for another 15 to 30 minutes, until the internal temperature of the meat is 125 degrees F.

Remove the roast from the oven and transfer it to a cutting board. Cover it tightly with aluminum foil and allow the meat to rest for 20 minutes. In the meantime, put the asparagus on a cookie sheet and toss with the oil and balsamic vinegar and the Grana Padano and bake at 350 for about five minutes.

HOW TO SERVE YOURSELF: Carve a big, juicy red slice for yourself and serve with horseradish sauce, jus, and asparagus.

HOW TO SERVE YOUR DOG: Carve some meat and cut into small pieces, then serve at room temperature in your puppy's best Sunday dinner bowl.

Fat Daisy's Inner-Strength Training

Take your dog for an after-dinner constitutional and see how different your neighborhood looks when the sun goes down.

Day 14

Inner-Beauty Thought for the Day:

There is no psychiatrist in the world like a puppy licking your face.

—BEN WILLIAMS

Breakfast: Yes I Am Green Eggs and Ham

Preheat the oven to 375 degrees F.

HERE'S WHAT YOU'LL NEED:
1/4 cup half and half
3 eggs
1/2 cup minced fresh herbs, such as
    parsley, rosemary, basil, and thyme
Salt
Freshly ground pepper (people
    portions only)
4 tablespoons Grana Padano
Sliced baked Virginia ham
2 tablespoons butter

HERE'S HOW YOU DO IT: Pour the half and half into a small skillet and place in the oven until it gets hot. When the cream is very hot, but not burning, pull the skillet out of the oven, crack the eggs into the hot cream, cover with herbs, salt, pepper (for humans only!), and cheese and put back in the oven until hot and bubbly. Meanwhile, fry up your favorite Virginia ham or ham steak in a skillet, using the butter, and serve alongside the shirred eggs.

HOW TO SERVE YOURSELF: Serve in the skillet with ham on the side.

HOW TO SERVE YOUR DOG: Cut up the ham and mix with one of the eggs in a bowl. Serve at room temperature.

Fat Daisy's Inner-Beauty Regimen

Get crafty and make something that your dog will enjoy. Learn how to knit and knit your puppy a sweater, or make your puppy a new toy. It feels good to get creative and make things for the people that you love, even if one sleeve turns out to be longer than the other.

Dinner: Inner-Peace Pot

This dish leaves you with a warm, peaceful feeling way down inside.

HERE'S WHAT YOU'LL NEED:
Salt
2 boneless chicken breasts, cut into
    bite-sized pieces
A little olive oil
2 cups chicken stock (16 ounces)
1/2 cup apple cider
2 peppercorns
1 whole clove
1 bay leaf
1 sweet potato, peeled and cut into
    bite-sized pieces
1 cup baby carrots
1 apple, peeled, cored, and cut into
    bite-sized pieces

HERE'S HOW YOU DO IT: Salt your chicken, then sauté in a little olive oil until lightly browned. Next, add the chicken stock and scrape the little brown bits off the bottom of the pan. These little bits add a lot of flavor to your sauce. Next, add the cider, peppercorns, clove, and bay leaf, cover, and bring to a boil. Lower the heat, add the vegetables and the apple, and simmer until tender, about 20 minutes. And remember, whoever gets the bay leaf gets a wish!

HOW TO SERVE YOURSELF: Spoon a little of each of the ingredients into a wide-rimmed soup bowl and drizzle with jus. Serve hot with a little fresh cracked pepper.

HOW TO SERVE YOUR DOG: Allow to cool to room temperate, then spoon into a bowl and cover with jus.

Fat Daisy's Inner-Strength Training

It's the last day, so sprint to the finish line by taking your puppy for a run, and then taking a nice, long, hot bubble bath together and congratulating your-selves on your healthy lifestyle.

Daisy's Bringing
Sexy Back

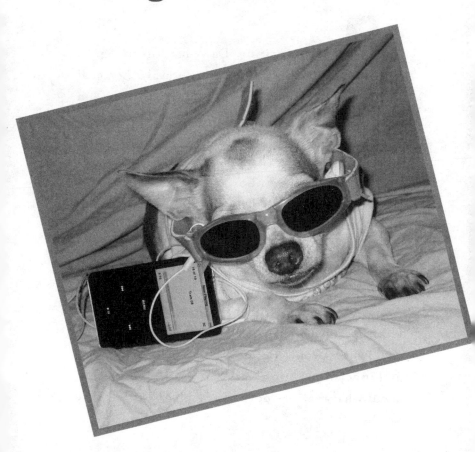

As of this writing, Daisy has lost five and a half pounds and is still working toward her goal weight with her signature strength of purpose. And while we have all accepted that Daisy is never going to be a teacup pocket pooch, or a glamorous Hollywood accessory dog, she is looking and feeling like the sexy bitch she was born to be. These days she can be found trotting through fields of clover with Elvis, Bert, and Buddha, and chasing Hamlet all over the house without the need for any medication or surgery. These days, she is still working toward being one size healthier, and hopes to become America's very first canine fitness guru. She has recently launched her own Web site, www.FatDaisy.com, where people and pets can get advice, recipes, and inner-beauty tips, and learn from one another about what they are doing to be the best that they can be.

And while Elvis never cared at all about Daisy's weight, and remained madly in love with her at any size, he is thrilled to be able to once again roll around on the floor in a puppy pile of joy with her.

So we are happy to report that Daisy, Elvis, Bert and Buddha, and Hamlet, and the two turtles, Liza and Jude, and the fourteen fish are all living happily ever after.

And so are Jason and I.

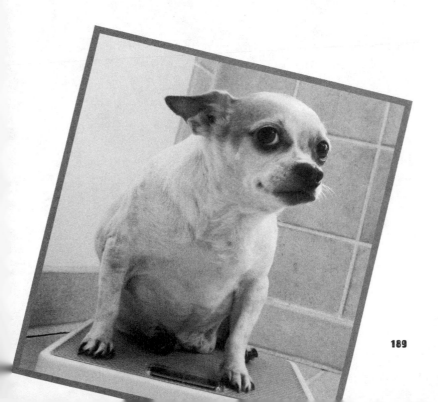